Updates in Foot and Ankle Arthritis

Editor

JEFFREY E. MCALISTER

CLINICS IN PODIATRIC MEDICINE AND SURGERY

www.podiatric.theclinics.com

Consulting Editor
THOMAS J. CHANG

October 2023 • Volume 40 • Number 4

ELSEVIER

1600 John F. Kennedy Boulevard • Suite 1800 • Philadelphia, Pennsylvania, 19103-2899

http://www.theclinics.com

CLINICS IN PODIATRIC MEDICINE AND SURGERY Volume 40, Number 4
October 2023 ISSN 0891-8422, ISBN-13: 978-0-443-18234-1

Editor: Megan Ashdown
Developmental Editor: Anita Chamoli

Clinics in Podiatric Medicine and Surgery (ISSN 0891-8422) is published quarterly by Elsevier Inc., 360 Park Avenue South, New York, NY 10010-1710. Months of issue are January, April, July, and October. Business and Editorial Offices: 1600 John F. Kennedy Blvd., Ste. 1800, Philadelphia, PA 19103-2899. Customer Service Office: 3251 Riverport Lane, Maryland Heights, MO 63043. Periodicals postage paid at New York, NY and additional mailing offices. Subscription prices are $329.00 per year for US individuals, $625.00 per year for US institutions, $100.00 per year for US students and residents, $405.00 per year for Canadian individuals, $754.00 for Canadian institutions, $490.00 for international individuals, $754.00 per year for international institutions, $100.00 per year for Canadian students/residents, and $220.00 per year for foreign students/residents. To receive student/resident rate, orders must be accompanied by name of affiliated institution, date of term, and the *signature* of program/residency coordinator on institution letterhead. Orders will be billed at individual rate until proof of status is received. Foreign air speed delivery is included in all *Clinics* subscription prices. All prices are subject to change without notice. POSTMASTER: Send address changes to *Clinics in Podiatric Medicine and Surgery*, Elsevier Health Sciences Division, Subscription Customer Service, 3251 Riverport Lane, Maryland Heights, MO 63043. **Customer Service: 1-800-654-2452 (US). From outside of the US, call 314-447-8871. Fax: 314-447-8029. E-mail: JournalsCustomerService-usa@elsevier.com (for print support); JournalsOnlineSupport-usa@elsevier.com (for online support).**

Reprints. For copies of 100 or more of articles in this publication, please contact the Commercial Reprints Department, Elsevier Inc., 360 Park Avenue South, New York, NY 10010-1710. Tel.: 212-633-3874; Fax: 212-633-3820; E-mail: reprints@elsevier.com.

Clinics in Podiatric Medicine and Surgery is covered in *MEDLINE/PubMed (Index Medicus)* and *EMBASE/Excerpta Medica.*

Contributors

CONSULTING EDITOR

THOMAS J. CHANG, DPM
Clinical Professor and Past Chairman, Department of Podiatric Surgery, CCPM Faculty,
The Podiatry Institute, Sonoma County Orthopedic/Podiatric Specialists, Santa Rosa,
California

EDITOR

JEFFREY E. MCALISTER, DPM, FACFAS
Fellowship-Trained, Program Director, Foot and Ankle Surgical Fellowship Program,
Phoenix Foot and Ankle Institute, Scottsdale, Arizona

AUTHORS

LANT ABERNATHY, DPM, AACFAS
Fellow, The CORE Institute Advanced Foot and Ankle Reconstruction Fellowship,
Phoenix, Arizona

JAY S. BADELL, DPM, AACFAS
Fellow, Florida Orthopedic Foot & Ankle Center, Sarasota, Florida

DOMINICK CASCIATO, DPM, AACFAS
Department of Orthopaedics, Fellow, Limb Preservation and Deformity Correction
Fellowship, University of Maryland School of Medicine, Baltimore, Maryland

ROBERT C. CLEMENTS, DPM, MS
JFK Medical Center Foot and Ankle Surgery Atlantis, Florida

ELIZABETH C. CONNOLLY, DPM
JFK Medical Center Foot and Ankle Surgery Atlantis, Florida

HELENE R. COOK, DPM, AACFAS
Fellow, Northern California Reconstructive Foot and Ankle Fellowship, Shasta
Orthopaedics and Sports Medicine, Redding, California

JAMES M. COTTOM, DPM, FACFAS
Florida Orthopedic Foot & Ankle Center, Sarasota, Florida

JASON GEORGE DEVRIES, DPM, FACFAS
Orthopedics and Sports Medicine, BayCare Clinic, Manitowoc, Wisconsin

KEEGAN A. DUELFER, DPM
Fellow, Foot and Ankle Surgical Fellowship Program, Phoenix Foot and Ankle Institute,
Scottsdale, Arizona

AMAR GULATI, DPM
Attending Physician, Progressive Feet, Arlington, Virginia

PETER D. HIGHLANDER, DPM, MS
Fellowship Director, The Reconstruction Institute, The Bellevue Hospital, Bellevue, Ohio

CHRISTOPER F. HYER, DPM, MS, FACFAS
Fellowship Co-Director, Advanced Foot and Ankle Reconstruction, Orthopedic Foot and Ankle Center, Worthington, Ohio

AMBER KAVANAGH, DPM, AACFAS
ACFAS Fellow, Hinsdale Orthopaedics (IBJI) Foot and Ankle Fellowship, Joliet, Illinois

KWASI Y. KWAADU, DPM, FACFAS
Chair, Department of Podiatric Surgery, Temple University Health Systems; Podiatric Surgical Residency, Assistant Director, Temple University Hospital, Clinical Associate Professor, Department of Surgery, Temple University School of Podiatric Medicine, Philadelphia, Pennsylvania

RYAN J. LERCH, DPM
Fellow, The Reconstruction Institute, The Bellevue Hospital, Bellevue, Ohio

CHANDLER LIGAS, DPM
Fellow, Foot and Ankle Surgery, Silicon Valley Reconstructive Foot and Ankle Fellowship, Mountain View, California

SARA MATEEN, DPM, AACFAS
Fellow, Foot and Ankle Deformity and Orthoplastics, Clinical Fellow, International Center of Limb Lengthening, Rubin Institute for Advanced Orthopedics, Baltimore, Maryland

JEFFREY E. MCALISTER, DPM, FACFAS
Fellowship-Trained, Program Director, Foot and Ankle Surgical Fellowship Program, Phoenix Foot and Ankle Institute, Scottsdale, Arizona

COLLIN MESSERLY, DPM, AACFAS
Attending Physician, Town Center Orthopedics, Ashburn, Virginia

JASON NOWAK, DPM, FACFAS
Fellowship Director, Northern California Reconstructive Foot and Ankle Fellowship, Shasta Orthopaedics and Sports Medicine, Redding, California

JACOB M. PERKINS, DPM, AACFAS
Post-Graduate Fellow, Orthopedic Foot and Ankle Center Advanced Foot and Ankle Reconstruction Fellowship, Worthington, Ohio

KYLE S. PETERSON, DPM, FACFAS
Fellowship-Trained, Board Certified Foot and Ankle Surgeon, Suburban Orthopaedics, Bartlett, Illinois

MARK A. PRISSEL, DPM, FACFAS
Fellowship-Trained, Board Certified Foot and Ankle Surgeon, Fellowship Director, Advanced Foot and Ankle Reconstruction, Orthopedic Foot and Ankle Center Advanced Foot and Ankle Reconstruction Fellowship, Worthington, Ohio

NILIN M. RAO, DPM, PhD, FACFAS
Board-Certified, Fellowship-Trained, Foot and Ankle Surgeon, Foot Specialists of Austin, Austin, Texas

BRANDON M. SCHARER, DPM, FACFAS
Orthopedics and Sports Medicine, BayCare Clinic, Green Bay, Wisconsin

RYAN T. SCOTT, DPM, FACFAS
Fellowship Director, The CORE Institute Advanced Foot and Ankle Reconstruction Fellowship, Phoenix, Arizona

JOSHUA A. SEBAG, DPM, FACFAS
Coastal Orthopaedic & Sports Medicine Center, Palm City, Florida

NOMAN A. SIDDIQUI, DPM, MHA
International Center of Limb Lengthening, Rubin Institute for Advanced Orthopedics, Director, Foot and Ankle Deformity Correction and Orthoplastics Fellowship, Chair, Division of Podiatry, Sinai and Northwest Hospital, Baltimore, Maryland

MATTHEW D. SORENSEN, DPM, FACFAS
OrthoIllinois, Chicago, Illinois

GARRET STRAND, DPM, AACFAS
Assistant Fellowship Director, Northern California Reconstructive Foot and Ankle Fellowship, Shasta Orthopaedics and Sports Medicine, Redding, California

EDGAR SY, DPM, AACFAS
Fellow, Weil Foot & Ankle Institute, Chicago, Illinois

STEVEN A. TOCCI, DPM, AACFAS
Fellow, The CORE Institute Advanced Foot and Ankle Reconstruction Fellowship, Phoenix, Arizona

CODY J. TOGHER, DPM, AACFAS
Joint Replacement Institute, Naples, Florida

VINCENT G. VACKETTA, DPM, AACFAS
Post-Graduate Fellow, Orthopedic Foot and Ankle Center Advanced Foot and Ankle Reconstruction Fellowship, Worthington, Ohio

JOSEPH R. WOLF, DPM, AACFAS
Fellow, Florida Orthopedic Foot & Ankle Center, Sarasota, Florida

JACOB WYNES, DPM, MS, FACFAS
Assistant Professor, Department of Orthopaedics, Program Director, Limb Preservation and Deformity Correction Fellowship, University of Maryland School of Medicine, Baltimore, Maryland

Contents

> First metatarsophalangeal joint (MPJ) arthrodesis procedures are a main-
> stay of forefoot surgery and are associated with high rates of patient sat-
> isfaction for addressing a multitude of first ray pathologic conditions. This
> procedure is often also used as a fallback option for the revision of poor
> outcomes after other surgical procedures involving the first ray. Despite
> its successes, there remain instances of complications that can develop
> after primary first MPJ arthrodesis. This article reviews first MPJ arthrod-
> esis as a procedure for revisional surgery of the first ray, and potential sur-
> gical options after failed primary first MPJ arthrodesis.

> Tarsometatarsal joint injuries can be painful and debilitating and are most
> commonly due to direct or indirect trauma. Posttraumatic arthritis is a well-
> known long-term complication, with incidence as high as 58%. Conserva-
> tive treatment options include shoe modifications, orthotic inserts, topical
> or oral anti-inflammatories, and intra-articular corticosteroid injections.
> There are various joint prep and fixation techniques reported in the litera-
> ture, many with positive clinical and radiographic outcomes. This article
> discusses nonoperative and operative management of posttraumatic tar-
> sometatarsal joint arthritis, reviews available literature, and includes the
> authors' tips and techniques.

> The objective of this article is to review the etiology and pathophysiology of
> Charcot neuroarthropathy as it contributes to the breakdown of the mid-
> foot. The article will also discuss the emerging techniques in minimally in-
> vasive surgery and how this is applied to Charcot reconstructive surgery as
> well as reflect on a newer thought processes to surgical intervention.

The newer generation total ankle arthroplasty constructs afford higher levels of long-term survivability, and for the first in the history of ankle arthroplasty procedures, results are comparable to arthrodesis. Much of the success hinges on appropriate patient selection. A comprehensive workup of the patient will allow selection of adjunctive procedures as well as allowing for the determination of single versus 2-stage deformity correction. With the continual addition of implants, it is important to understand the specialization and indications that are assigned to certain models because this will help in selecting the most appropriate implant for any given patient.

Avascular necrosis (AVN) of the talus is a difficult pathology to treat. Patient-specific factors such as functional status, comorbidities should be considered. Previous standard care for talar AVN was centered around arthrodesis procedures and loss of motion about the joints of the rearfoot and ankle. With the advent of 3D printed talar implants, patients are afforded an option to maintain ankle joint motion. Literature is limited due to the recent development of total talus replacement (TTR) technology. This article aims to review literature, surgical techniques, and pearls to better help foot and ankle surgeons treat cases of talar AVN.

Ankle arthritis is a disabling disease pattern resulting in pain and dysfunction ultimately leading to a reduction in quality of life. Unlike more common arthritides of the knee and hip, ankle arthritis is unique in its presentation with an earlier onset of end-stage disease and an etiology, which is most-commonly posttraumatic in nature. Through continued research and design, improvements have continued to be made as newer generation implants are developed. This article discusses the considerations for revision total ankle replacement based on the current revision options and a treatment algorithm developed by the lead author.

The supramalleolar osteotomy (SMO) is a joint-preserving surgical procedure that allows realignment of the ankle joint in severe deformity secondary to arthritis. This osteotomy realigns the mechanical axis to provide better weight distribution through the ankle joint. With an aligned mechanical axis, the overloaded asymmetric ankle joint will shift toward the preserved joint area in a valgus or varus ankle joint. The SMO also can be used via a staged approach to correct severe deformity in an end-stage arthritic ankle before total ankle arthroplasty to optimize the implant's longevity and improve overall functional outcomes.

CLINICS IN PODIATRIC MEDICINE AND SURGERY

THE CLINICS ARE AVAILABLE ONLINE!
Access your subscription at:
www.theclinics.com

Foreword

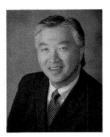

Thomas J. Chang, DPM
Consulting Editor

In the United States, 24% of all adults, or 58.5 million people, have arthritis. It is a leading cause of work disability, with annual costs for medical care and lost earnings of $303.5 billion. The most common form of arthritis is osteoarthritis. Approximately 80% to 90% of individuals older than 65 years have evidence of radiographic primary osteoarthritis.

Arthritis is a condition we cannot avoid. In any Foot and Ankle office, arthritis is even more common than Plantar Fasciitis. Some patients will suffer from a flatfoot or cavus foot condition and even common tendonitis, yet as a condition of reaching older age, everyone will suffer from a form of arthritis.

I felt it was time to revisit new thoughts and discussions on the treatment options for common arthritic conditions of the foot and ankle. Since the last issue on arthritis in 2010, we have embraced new biologics and implants with updated techniques and perspectives. The state-of-the-art back then has been studied carefully, and we now know the successes and downfalls of those previous concepts. Over the past 5 years, custom and patient-specific implants can now be considered in difficult cases where there were minimal options in the past. It is an exciting time.

Dr McAlister has shown a passion in this topic area throughout the years. He is a practitioner with tremendous experience in surgical management of these deformities. He also shares valuable insight into his work experiences with words of wisdom as we all navigate the world of social media and private practice. It is invaluable to hear his personal insights, especially for the younger practitioner.

Clin Podiatr Med Surg 40 (2023) xiii–xiv
https://doi.org/10.1016/j.cpm.2023.06.015
0891-8422/23/© 2023 Published by Elsevier Inc.

I know you will find this issue valuable.

Thomas J. Chang, DPM
Sonoma County Orthopedic/
Podiatric Specialists
3536 Mendocino Avenue, Suite 300B
Santa Rosa, CA 95403, USA

E-mail address:
thomaschang14@comcast.net

Preface

Growth in Private Practice

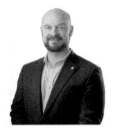

Jeffrey E. McAlister, DPM, FACFAS
Editor

I have had the honor and pleasure of piecemealing together some of the brightest and most talented authors in the field for this *Clinics in Podiatric Medicine and Surgery* issue. I want to thank my mentors and Thomas Chang for the opportunity to help edit and coauthor this issue.

My growth in this field has allowed me to hustle and bustle through a large orthopedic group and grow both professionally and personally. I also had the opportunity to expand in the private foot and ankle sector, which in my humble opinion is not completely dead. I wanted to write a short preface on my tips and pearls to expanding your footprint and getting a grasp on the fears that most residents, fellows, and young practitioners have about private practice.

First, you don't need a million dollars to start a practice. Believe it or not, despite what multiple practice "consultants" will tell you, start-up costs are less than what is assumed. Focus on location, location, location as your main priority—a similar concept as with any business. Make it easy for your patients to travel and find you. The most worthwhile out-of-pocket costs at first are your staff and team. Spend good money on a team that understands your vision and growth potential. Most of the hard goods in your office, just to get you started, are and can be placed on a credit card or paid for on an invoice, which means you don't need up-front cash (eg, exam tables, computers, office supplies, and durable medical equipment). These items are typically net-ninety or can be paid for on a revolving basis. The office space is obviously important and should look the part. One should spend quality dollars on quality products and equipment. Ask yourself: *What would YOU want to be treated with?*

Second, marketing is of utmost importance in the early years. Spend money to make money. I am no businessman. I am a physician like most readers, but please understand that patients must find you and learn about your niches and specialties. This does not rely *solely* on word of mouth but also on the physician's online presence and ability to differentiate among peers. I took many nights to create Web pages that allowed readers to learn about various topics and blogs that were targeted at specific disease processes and pathologies. This bumps up your search engine optimization (which is still important) and Google awareness. This is soft marketing, in my opinion, but hard marketing is the standard door-to-door marketing strategy. Believe it or not, this is still critical and crucial to growth, even today. My staff will visit urgent cares, primary care physicians, and chiropractors and get the word out about the team and patient care. So do not assume that people will just find you in the Yellow Pages; you must go get it and work for it.

Last, your office staff and in-office flow and energy must reflect your work and patient care. I know it's corny, but my mentors told me: Treat everyone like family and you'll never lose. I still carry that thought process in my everyday clinic and life because it's true. It comes down to training your staff on the treatment of patients, the music you play in the office, and the complimentary smiles that are required upon patients exiting. Asking the patient if they have any questions. Confirming their follow-up appointment with an appointment card. Giving out my cell phone for patient questions if needed. Spending time with every patient like it was the only patient of the day. There is something to be said about concierge medicine, and if you can practice that and be a great surgeon, you'll win and win big. My parting words revolve around patient reviews and focusing on obtaining quality and real words from your patients. It's my practice growth calculator and everyday practice builder.

Being an editor for this issue of *Clinics in Podiatric Medicine and Surgery* has been an excellent source of pride and enjoyment, as we impart knowledge on arthritic conditions in the foot and ankle as well as theories on revision cases and complexities seen by all. I hope that each reader takes away a pearl from each article and can treat all arthritic patients like family.

Jeffrey E. McAlister, DPM, FACFAS
Foot and Ankle Surgical Fellowship Program
Phoenix Foot and Ankle Institute
Scottsdale, AZ, USA

E-mail address:
Jeff.mcalister@phoenixfai.com

The First Metatarsophalangeal Joint
Updates on Revision Arthrodesis and Malunions

Joshua A. Sebag, DPM, FACFAS[a],*, Robert C. Clements, DPM, MS[b],
Cody J. Togher, DPM, AACFAS[c], Elizabeth C. Connolly, DPM[b]

KEYWORDS

- Hallux rigidus • Hallux valgus • Arthrodesis • Fusion
- First metatarsophalangeal joint • Revision surgery • Forefoot salvage
- Critically sized defects

KEY POINTS

- Deformity correction is pivotal for successful outcomes. Malalignment may increase the chances of nonunion secondary to imbalance of mechanical forces across the fusion mass.
- Proper debridement of fusion mass surfaces is essential. Medullary bone should be exposed on all surfaces to ensure adequate vascular supply to the fusion.
- Autograft should be used when appropriate: Either in isolation or in combination with structural allografts when addressing osseous defects and first ray shortening.
- Use constructs that are rigid enough to prevent unwanted motion across the fusion mass, especially when using structural implants that have a tendency to move or shorten during the postoperative healing period. This is of particular importance in any revision arthrodesis attempt.
- Advanced imaging, namely MRI and or computed tomography scans should be considered in revision metatarsophalangeal joint arthrodesis.

INTRODUCTION

First metatarsophalangeal joint (MPJ) arthrodesis has a high degree of utility as the primary surgical option in the treatment of first ray pathologic condition and can be used as a salvage option for failed first ray procedures. From a biomechanical perspective, first MPJ arthrodesis provides correction of deformity and elimination of painful arthritis, as well as improving the weight-bearing function of the first ray.[1] This

[a] Coastal Orthopaedic & Sports Medicine Center, 5158 Southwest Anhinga Avenue, Palm City, FL 34990, USA; [b] JFK Medical Center Foot and Ankle Surgery Residency Program; [c] Joint Replacement Institute, 3466 Pine Ridge RD, Suite A, Naples, FL 34109, USA
* Corresponding author.
E-mail address: Sebag.Josh@gmail.com

Clin Podiatr Med Surg 40 (2023) 569–580
https://doi.org/10.1016/j.cpm.2023.05.002
0891-8422/23/© 2023 Elsevier Inc. All rights reserved.

provides improved propulsion of the ankle joint complex allowing for increased single limb support and decreased step width during ambulation.[2] Because of a patient's ability to retain the biomechanical advantage of the first ray after undergoing first MPJ arthrodesis, the procedure has historically been recommended for more active populations as a definitive surgical treatment option.

In addition to the relative maintenance of a physiologic gait, there remains a high degree of patient satisfaction concerning function and activity after undergoing first MPJ arthrodesis. Da Cunha and colleagues in 2019 retrospectively assessed 50 patients through a prospective registry who underwent first MPJ arthrodesis. They found that patients returned to 44.6% of their physical activities within 6 months, obtained maximal participation in 88.6% of activities, and had an overall satisfaction rating of 96%.[3] More recently, a study by Dayton and colleagues was performed assessing patient-reported activity following first MPJ arthrodesis. Out of 60 subjects, 95% reported that loss of first MPJ motion did not affect their ability to perform normal daily activities, and 93% expressed subjective success with the surgical outcome. The authors also identified patient-reported increases in recreational activities such as running, biking, golfing, yoga, and hiking; in summation, 97% of patients conveyed satisfaction with their ability to return to recreational activities after undergoing first MPJ arthrodesis.[4]

Further rationale in favor of first MPJ arthrodesis is the ability to provide a significant amount of deformity correction when addressing hallux valgus deformities. In 2006, Cronin and colleagues performed a retrospective study, which assessed first intermetatarsal angle (IMA) correction following first MPJ arthrodesis. They demonstrated a relatively high mean preoperative IMA of 16.65°, corrected to 8.67° at final follow-up.[5] Feilmeie and colleagues[6,7] in 2014 assessed the first IMA of patients undergoing primary first MPJ arthrodesis, reporting an overall correction rate of 5.44° and degree of correction correlating to the magnitude of the preoperative IMA.

Success rates for primary first MPJ arthrodesis are relatively high because the procedure eliminates the painful arthrosis experienced by patients with hallux limitus or rigidus and leads to low reported revision rates. Roukis and colleagues[8] in 2011 performed a systematic review of 2656 first MPJ fusions and demonstrated that union rates with modern techniques are approximately 94.6%, and only 32.7% of those experiencing nonunion as being symptomatic. Although primary first MPJ arthrodesis is a relatively successful procedure, revision cases can be fraught with challenges, especially when addressing bone loss and complex deformities. The nuances of revision MPJ fusion are numerous. With an increase in active and elder populations and a tendency of failed procedures to end in first ray fusions, revision first MPJ arthrodesis is likely to remain an important tool of the modern foot surgeon. This article will discuss recent updates regarding revision first MPJ arthrodesis with a focus on painful malunions, nonunions, arthroplasty conversion, as well as treatment strategies for complex first ray deformities with significant segmental bone loss and critically sized defects (CSDs).

UPDATES FOR PRIMARY FIRST METATARSOPHALANGEAL JOINT ARTHRODESIS

Joint debridement via cup and cone reaming can be used, and it can assist with ease of joint positioning in all 3 planes. It is important to consider abnormal hallux valgus positions greater than 20° before definitive fixation because this has been identified as an independent risk factor for nonunion.[9] Eccentric reaming techniques can aid in deformity correction during joint preparation.[10] As described by Consul and Hyer, this technique involves the eccentric placement of reaming guidewires, perpendicular to the interphalangeal joint (IPJ) of the hallux. This facilitates the correction of hallux valgus and interphalangeus deformities while also preserving the cup and cone shape of the phalanx base and metatarsal head. Ancillary sesamoidectomy can be performed if metatarsosesamoid pathologic condition exists. A recent cadaveric study performed by Togher and colleagues[11] described a transarticular approach for sesamoid removal through a standard dorsal incision, preventing the necessity for additional, superfluous, plantar, or medial incisions.

With improvements in joint preparation techniques, positioning, and fixation constructs, authors have advocated for earlier weight-bearing protocols. In 2014, Dayton and colleagues[12] retrospectively assessed early ambulation with various fixation constructs in 47 patients following primary first MPJ arthrodesis reporting a 100% union rate. More recently, Elgut and colleagues retrospectively assessed patients following first MPJ arthrodesis. Subjects in this study began early weight-bearing at 5 days postoperatively in a controlled ankle motion (CAM) walker boot with a first ray cutout, demonstrating a 97.4% union rate.[13] Abben and colleagues[14] in 2018 reported similar outcomes with immediate postoperative weight-bearing demonstrating a 96% union rate. Based on these studies, early weight-bearing can be initiated safely following primary first MPJ arthrodesis when proper joint preparation techniques and rigid fixation constructs are used.

COMPLICATIONS OF PRIMARY FIRST METATARSOPHALANGEAL JOINT ARTHRODESIS AND ARTHROPLASTY LEADING TO REVISION

Various complications can occur following primary first MPJ arthrodesis. Based on a large systematic review by Roukis in 2017, the most common complications included malunion, nonunion,[8] and painful hardware requiring removal. This was supported by another study performed by Gaudin and colleagues in 2018. This report identified the most common reasons for reoperation were secondary to painful hardware, nonunion, malunion, metatarsalgia or claw toe deformity, and hallux IPJ joint disorders.[15] If painful hardware is present postoperatively, hardware removal can be considered once there is confirmation of radiographic union at the arthrodesis site. The authors of this article think as though this is not achieved until at least 6 months postsurgery. Cases of nonunion and malunion are frequently associated with inadequate deformity correction or fixation, which can be prevented with proper joint preparation, positioning, and rigid internal fixation constructs as discussed with primary first MPJ arthrodesis.[9]

Similar to arthrodesis procedures, failure of first MPJ arthroplasties can occur due to instability or malposition of the first MPJ. Arthrofibrosis, synovitis, and periprosthetic stress fractures might also warrant conversion to arthrodesis. These complications can be further magnified in active populations who place greater amounts of stress across the first MPJ during dynamic activity. Stone and colleagues assessed the long-term outcomes of first MPJ arthroplasty versus arthrodesis. At final followup, they found that pain relief and overall satisfaction was superior in the arthrodesis group, and that most of the arthroplasty patients were eventually converted to a first MPJ arthrodesis. This study demonstrates that first MPJ arthrodesis can be advantageous in reducing pain, preventing multiple surgeries and is useful when revising failed first MPJ arthroplasty with improved long-term patient outcomes scores.[16] Conversion from first MPJ arthroplasty to arthrodesis is a mainstay of first MPJ revision surgery; however, bone loss and shortening of the first ray may complicate the procedure and necessitate structural bone graft to restore anatomical position and prevent the subsequent transfer forces to lesser metatarsal heads.

REVISION AND SALVAGE FIRST METATARSOPHALANGEAL JOINT ARTHRODESIS

Failed primary procedures of the first ray may pose challenges, especially in the presence of avascular bone and CSDs. Complications after revisional surgery of the first MPJ occur more frequently than primary procedures, further convoluting circumstances. This was exhibited in a study by Prat and colleagues[17] in 2022. Their findings demonstrated a 41% complication rate with 19% nonunion, of which 9% required additional revisional surgery. The authors also identified risk factors for complications requiring reoperation to include diabetes mellitus, tobacco use, and "in situ" joint preparation techniques. This suggests the value of preoperative evaluation and management of patient comorbidities as well as the practice of proper joint preparation techniques. Furthermore, any underlying deformities or biomechanical instability should be assessed. This is particularly important in cases with coinciding forefoot deformities of the lesser rays. As demonstrated by Thier and colleagues,[18] recurrent dislocations, lesser toe deformities, metatarsus adductus, and cavus foot types were identified as risk factors for revisional surgery in primary first ray procedures. This study also supported the preoperative management of patient-specific medical comorbidities such as diabetes mellitus and tobacco use, which they identified as independent risk factors for revision after first-ray procedures.

An alternative to revision of first MPJ arthrodesis includes hardware removal and/or arthroplasty conversion. These procedures may be considered for select patient populations including older sedentary patients with low physical demands, or those who remain at a high risk for nonunion. A 2010 study performed by Hope and colleagues retrospectively assessed patients who underwent either arthroplasty conversion, secondary arthrodesis, or hardware removal after failed primary first MPJ fusion. They found that patients with nonunion who received isolated hardware removal or arthroplasty conversion expressed unsatisfactory outcomes leading to a 36% chance of additional revision surgery.[19] In contrast, a more recent study performed by Gaudin and colleagues investigated intermediate-term results after primary first MPJ fusion procedures. Using American Orthopaedic Foot and Ankle Society (AOFAS) and Short Form-12 scores, they found that patients had a higher overall satisfaction with isolated hardware removal compared with repeated arthrodesis in the setting of nonunion.[15] There remains a paucity of literature investigating the outcomes of revisional fusion versus hardware removal with or without conversion to arthroplasty, and it remains up to the surgeon to guide the patient and work together to perform a realistic treatment plan in each specific situation.

FIXATION FOR SALVAGE AND REVISION FIRST METATARSOPHALANGEAL JOINT ARTHRODESIS

Fixation for revision and salvage first MPJ arthrodesis typically consists of a well-contoured dorsal plate or a commercially available revision plate, which typically consists of a longer variation of primary plates, and may possess flanges that wrap around the bone allowing for internal compression and the ability to secure interposed grafts. Analogous to primary first MPJ arthrodesis, excessive extension is discouraged and only a minimal amount of dorsal plate bending is required (typically $0°-5°$) due to the inherent conical configuration of the proximal phalanx.[20] Both locking and nonlocking plates can be considered; however, in cases of poor bone stock or significant osseous defects, locking plates are advantageous. Following temporary plate placement, additional crossing cannulated screws can be added for compression and to secure grafts. Dual-plating techniques have been recently described because some authors argue that a single dorsal plate is not ideally positioned on the tension side of the joint and plantar plating is not a viable option. Typically, the addition of a medial plate is used to prevent plantar gapping while securing both the graft and arthrodesis site. In 2015, Bei and colleagues[21] retrospectively assessed 11 revision first MPJ arthrodesis cases using bone graft and dual-plating fixation demonstrating a 90.9% union rate at an average time till union of 10.7 weeks with restoration of first ray length averaging 11 mm. **Fig. 1** demonstrates a case of bilateral first MPJ pathologic condition treated with revision arthrodesis using a biplanar plate construct. The procedures were performed unilaterally on separate dates.

CORRECTION OF SYMPTOMATIC MALUNION DEFORMITIES FOLLOWING PRIMARY FIRST METATARSOPHALANGEAL JOINT ARTHRODESIS

One of the primary reasons for performing revision first MPJ arthrodesis is malposition. Roukis and colleagues found that the average malunion rate following first MPJ arthrodesis was 6.1%. A further investigation by the authors identified that the vast majority of which were secondary to dorsal malalignment, followed by valgus overrotation.[8] Malunion has been identified as one of the leading risk factors for nonunion when performing arthrodesis of many joints about the midfoot and forefoot.[9,22] In cases of symptomatic malunion following first MPJ arthrodesis, successful patient outcomes can be achieved with hardware removal and corrective osteotomies based on the specific deformity present. Gaudin and colleagues[15] discovered that 8% of patients went onto malunion following primary first MPJ arthrodesis. If an ancillary osteotomy is necessary to perform in conjunction with arthrodesis, it is imperative to identify and target the dominant plane of deformity. In his early research, Paley defined the concept of the center of rotation of angulation as any point that leads to collinear realignment of the bone axes when the angulation correction axis passes through that point. When applying these principles, correction of malunion about the first MPJ can be outlined by the "Osteotomy Rules" as discussed by Coughlin, Paley, Mashima and colleagues.[23–25]

Anatomic sagittal plane alignment can be confirmed when the distal pulp of the Hallux is resting roughly 2 mm from the weight-bearing surface.[4] Additionally, the hallux IPJ should be aligned perpendicular to the long axis of the first ray. Sagittal plane malunions can be revised with hardware removal and either joint resection or osteotomies performed at the apex of the deformity. A plantar-flexed malunion

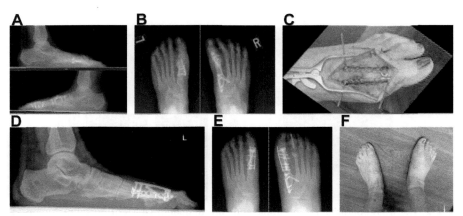

Fig. 1. (*A–F*) Preoperative imaging of bilateral first MPJ pathology (*A–B*) treated with revisional surgery in the form of MPJ arthrodesis (*C–F*).

increases plantar hallux pressure, especially during the propulsive phase of gait. This can lead to subsequent unsteady gait, adjacent joint arthritis due to abnormal distribution of ground reactive forces, and plantar wounds. Moberg or reverse Moberg osteotomies can be performed distal to the base of hallux. Plantarflexed malunions combined with significant residual hallux abductus interphalangeus can be addressed with multiplanar wedge osteotomies, as described by Hunt and colleagues.[26]

Other potential surgical options for dorsiflexed malunions of the first MPJ include crescentic osteotomies or trapezoidal osteotomies. Regardless of which osteotomy is selected, it is important to remember Paley's Osteotomy second rule.[24] Cullen and colleagues[27] in 2005 exhibited the effects of an opening wedge osteotomy of the proximal phalanx to revise malunion after first MPJ arthrodesis. **Fig. 2** demonstrates a case of a dorsal malunion of a first MPJ fusion treated secondarily via takedown osteotomy and corrective arthrodesis. In contrast to uniplanar deformities, multiplanar malunions often require a through-and-through osteotomy to achieve correct anatomical positioning in multiple cardinal body planes. Execution of this osteotomy requires thoughtful planning as to prevent excessive shortening of the first ray. When a short first ray is present in conjunction to malpositioning, bone grafting may be necessary to treat residual shortening, restore length, and to reestablish anatomical alignment.

CONVERSION FROM FIRST METATARSOPHALANGEAL JOINT ARTHROPLASTY TO ARTHRODESIS

Many complications can develop after first MPJ joint arthroplasty; however, one that can notably complicate revisional surgery and conversion to arthrodesis is the considerable amount of shortening the first ray can endure. Although an attempt to preserve length is made during joint-replacement procedures, a substantial amount of bone resection is required to make way for implants. Additionally, periprosthetic bone is likely of poor quality over time. If unaddressed, shortening can potentiate biomechanical imbalances that alter the dynamics of the metatarsal parabola. Depending on the degree of the remaining osseous defect, distraction arthrodesis may be warranted. A recent systematic review by Attia and colleagues analyzed autografts harvested from the calcaneus, proximal tibia, and distal tibial, and identified an overall complication

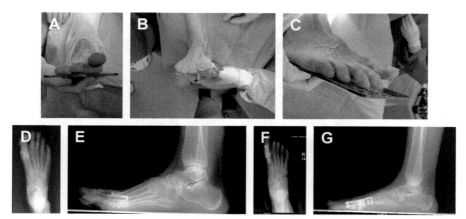

Fig. 2. (*A–D*) Preoperative radiographic and clinical images (*A–D*) of dorsal malunion of a first MPJ arthrodesis treated surgically with hardware removal and corrective osteotomy (*E, F, G*).

rate of 6.8%. This is relatively low when compared with the 19.3% that has traditionally been observed with iliac crest autograft.[28,29] Although other studies have substantiated the low risk of complications associated with the harvest of calcaneal autograft, they are typically limited to accommodating for defects of 1 to 2 cm.[28,30] Although it is rare to have defects of the first MPJ greater than 2 cm, this would call for the use of iliac crest autografts or available bulk allograft material.[31]

Allografts, especially when used in combination with bone marrow aspirate (BMA) or other autograft substrates, can be used as an alternative method for restoring first ray length while avoiding donor site complications. Luk and colleagues retrospectively reviewed revision first MPJ arthrodesis demonstrating interpositional allograft. Their results exhibited an 87% union rate with high patient satisfaction.[32] Similarly, Burke and colleagues[33] retrospectively assessed revision first MPJ arthrodesis using a patellar wedge interposition structural allograft with a 94.7% union rate with good or excellent outcomes. Overall, it seems that the size of the defect seems to dictate the appropriate selection of bone grafting when converting failed first MPJ arthroplasty to arthrodesis. In 2013 Garras and colleagues[31] exhibited high rates of fusion and functional scores for first MPJ hemiarthroplasty conversion to arthrodesis. **Fig. 3** demonstrate a case failed first MPJ hemiarthroplasty treated surgically with distraction arthrodesis using a combination of structural allograft and cancellous calcaneal autograft.

ADDRESSING SIGNIFICANT SEGMENTAL BONE LOSS

Unique surgical strategies must be implemented at times when addressing more complex, larger segmental first ray defects. Lamm and colleagues recently published a case report involving avascular necrosis and extensive segmental bone loss affecting the first metatarsal head, successfully treated with gradual medializing bone transport of the second metatarsal. After 12 months of follow-up, the authors were able to maintain the first ray position and length with no clinically significant complications, allowing for a pain-free return to activity.[34] Masquelet techniques have also been explored for extensive segmental bone loss as reported in a 2018 study by Liu and colleagues.

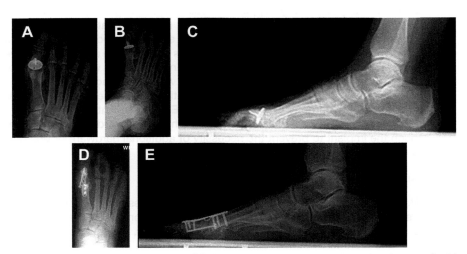

Fig. 3. (*A–E*) Preoperative imaging of failed first MPJ hemiarthroplasty (*A–C*) treated with distraction arthrodesis of the first MPJ (*D–E*).

In this case series, 11 patients were identified with first ray defects varying between 3 and 6 cm in length. Following the initial procedure, the authors performed a staged reconstruction of the residual osseous defect with the placement of antibiotic impregnated cement spacer, followed by subsequent arthrodesis with iliac cancellous bone graft and plate fixation during a tertiary surgery. All cases were successful after 11 months follow-up, defined by complete osseous union, lack of any significant complications, and acceptable functional outcomes.[35] In situations where massive defects or significant infection is present, consideration of partial first ray amputation with prosthesis may be necessary.

FUTURE CONSIDERATIONS

When substantial osseous defects and shortening of the first ray are associated with supplemental compromise of the arterial supply to osseous structures, this can leave few options for treating physicians; fortunately, recent advancements in 3D printing, patient-specific instrumentation, and patient-specific implants have expanded those options. Advanced imaging can help surgeons identify areas of avascular bone that may require resection, and these imaging modalities can be conveniently used to assist with patient-specific cutting guides to resect the appropriate amounts of necrotic bone without excessive shortening and worsening of osseous voids. These studies can be further used to help generate patient-specific surgical plans and implants consisting of gyroid, lattice, or truss-like structures. These designs allow for both osseous ingrowth between scaffolds, as well as ongrowth along the supporting metallic structures when the porous areas of the implant are filled with autologous bone graft.

Although this category of implant was originally used in spinal surgery, it has recently been described for the treatment of CSDs about the foot and ankle.[36] Although there remains a paucity of literature investigating the use of these patient-specific implants for CSDs of the first ray, there are several case studies that demonstrate their benefits.[37,38] Most recently, Hollawell and Coleman documented a report of 2 separate cases using defect-spanning custom implants in revisional first MPJ arthrodesis with satisfactory results after 14 to 20 months of follow-up.[39] Although it may still be too early to directly support the use of these implants, the authors of this article anticipate that future research and FDA recommendations will increase the use of patient-specific implants in foot and ankle surgery, including revisional first MPJ procedures with CSDs. **Fig. 4**A–D demonstrates preoperative and postoperative AP and lateral radiographs of a failed first MPJ primary arthrodesis with avascular necrosis of the proximal phalanx and metatarsal head. A custom made, gyroid-shaped cage was developed and an associated preoperative plan generated off weight-bearing computed tomography (CT) imaging (**Fig. 4**E). The implant and design were created in an attempt to resect all nonviable bone while also providing points of fixation through the implant to prevent the necessity of additional hardware or potential galvanic corrosion.

DISCUSSION

First MPJ arthrodesis has a high degree of utility for addressing a variety of first ray disorders and as a revision and salvage procedure. This procedure has numerous benefits for patients including relief of pain and deformity, durable lifelong lasting correction, and restoration of normal function, which results in relatively high patient satisfaction. In instances of malunion following primary first MPJ arthrodesis, deformity correction can be addressed with corrective osteotomies. If revision or salvage

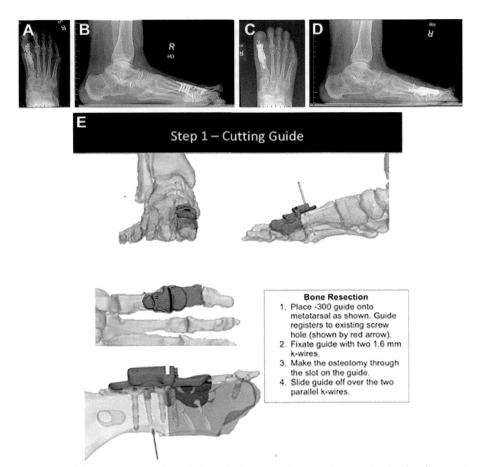

Fig. 4. (*A–E*) Preoperative CT renderings Including AP (*A*) and Lateral (*B*) of a first MPJ nonunion treated with patient-specific implant (*C–D*). Image 4E demonstrating patient-specific plan.

first MPJ arthrodesis is indicated, it is important to consider that there are higher complication rates when compared with primary procedures. In salvage cases with moderate loss of structural bone integrity, significant first ray shortening can be addressed with bone grafting. For larger segmental bone loss, unique strategies must be implemented including distraction osteogenesis, bone transport, and Masquelet techniques. If severe bone loss (area of abnormality) or deep infection persists, or when risks outweigh benefits, partial first ray amputation with prosthesis may be considered as a final resort.

CLINICS CARE POINTS

- Proper positioning is imperative during primary first MPJ arthrodesis. An improperly positioned fusion can lead to iatrogenic deformities and is one of the leading causes for nonunion and dysfunction. In cases of severe deformity (IMA >20)?, eccentric reaming techniques can be called on to reduce deformities while performing synchronous joint preparation.

- Careful joint preparation and attention to coinciding deformities should be observed during revision cases. Revision surgery and arthrodesis of the first MPJ has higher rates of nonunion compared with primary procedures. Failure to address simultaneous deformities and inadequate joint preparation techniques can further propagate nonunion and poor outcomes.

- Advanced imaging, namely MRI and CT scans, often reveal information, which may guide the treating surgeon and positively affect decision-making.

- Structural bone grafting can be practical when addressing multiplanar deformities with first ray shortening present. Harvest of calcaneal autograft is associated with relatively low rates of complications but only accommodates for defects up to 1 to 2 cm. Additionally, synthetic orthobiologics, although convenient, may not be necessary. The authors think autologous tissues may readily account for all graft needs. In the event of larger defects, allograft bone or iliac crest may be warranted.

- For exceptionally sized defects, or CSDs, newer options exist in the form of 3D printed metallic scaffolds. Although small case studies and reports have demonstrated satisfactory outcomes, further research is warranted to promote their benefits. This may become a reliable fallback option for tertiary revisions in the future.

DISCLOSURE

Dr J.A. Sebag is a consultant for Medartis, Vilex, CrossRoads, and ODI. No financial conflicts of interest exist and there are no funding sources for all authors.

REFERENCES

1. DeFrino PF, Brodsky JW, Pollo FE, et al. First metatarsophalangeal arthrodesis: a clinical, pedobarographic and gait analysis study. Foot Ankle Int 2002;23(6): 496–502.
2. Brodsky JW, Baum BS, Pollo FE, et al. Prospective gait analysis in patients with first metatarsophalangeal joint arthrodesis for hallux rigidus. Foot Ankle Int 2007;28(2):162–5.
3. Da Cunha RJ, MacMahon A, Jones MT, et al. Return to sports and physical activities after first metatarsophalangeal joint arthrodesis in young patients. Foot Ankle Int 2019 Jul;40(7):745–52.
4. Dayton M, Dayton P, Togher CJ, et al. What do patients report regarding their real-world function following triplane metatarsophalangeal joint arthrodesis for hallux valgus? J Foot Ankle Surg 2022.
5. Cronin JJ, Limbers JP, Kutty S, et al. Intermetatarsal angle after first metatarsophalangeal joint arthrodesis for hallux valgus. Foot Ankle Int 2006;27(2):104–9.
6. Feilmeier M, Dayton P, Wienke JC Jr. Reduction of intermetatarsal angle after first metatarsophalangeal joint arthrodesis in patients with hallux valgus. J Foot Ankle Surg 2014;53(1):29–31.
7. Dayton P, Feilmeier M, Hunziker B, et al. Reduction of the intermetatarsal angle after first metatarsal phalangeal joint arthrodesis: a systematic review. J Foot Ankle Surg 2014;53(5):620–3.
8. Roukis TS. Nonunion after arthrodesis of the first metatarsal-phalangeal joint: a systematic review. J Foot Ankle Surg 2011;50(6):710–3.
9. Weigelt L, Redfern J, Heyes GJ, et al. Risk factors for nonunion after first metatarsophalangeal joint arthrodesis with a dorsal locking plate and compression

screw construct: correction of hallux valgus Is key. J Foot Ankle Surg 2021;60(6): 1179–83.

10. Consul D. and Hyer CF. Eccentric reaming for first metatarsophalangeal joint fusion to address hallux interphalangeal joint position: technique guide and tips, *J Foot Ankle Surg*, 2022, In press.

11. Togher CJ, Vacketta VG, Thompson JM, et al. Sesamoid excision during first metatarsophalangeal joint arthrodesis via a transarticular approach: a cadaveric study. Foot Ankle Surg: Techniques, Reports, & Cases 2022;2(3).

12. Dayton P, McCall A. Early weightbearing after first metatarsophalangeal joint arthrodesis: a retrospective observational case analysis. J Foot Ankle Surg 2004;43(3):156–9.

13. Elgut D, Levin JS, Beth Z, et al. Analysis of fusion rates in patients undergoing 1st metatarsal phalangeal arthrodesis utilizing crossed compression screws w/dorsal neutralization plate & early weight bearing. Orthoped Rheumatol Open Access J 2016;3(5):1–4.

14. Abben KW, Sorensen MD, Waverly BJ. Immediate weightbearing after first metatarsophalangeal joint arthrodesis with screw and locking plate fixation: a short-term review. J Foot Ankle Surg 2018;57(4):771–5.

15. Gaudin G, Coillard JY, Augoyard M, et al, French Association of Foot Surgery (AFCP). Incidence and outcomes of revision surgery after first metatarsophalangeal joint arthrodesis: multicenter study of 158 cases. Orthop Traumatol Surg Res 2018;104(8):1221–6.

16. Stone OD, Ray R, Thomson CE, et al. Long-term follow-up of arthrodesis vs total joint arthroplasty for hallux rigidus. Foot Ankle Int 2017;38(4):375–80.

17. Prat D, Haghverdian BA, Pridgen EM, et al. High complication rates following revision first metatarsophalangeal joint arthrodesis: a retrospective analysis of 79 cases. Arch Orthop Trauma Surg 2023;143(4):1799–807.

18. Thier ZT, Seymour Z, Gonzalez TA, et al. Hallux valgus deformities: preferred surgical repair techniques and all-cause revision rates. Foot Ankle Spec 2021;25.

19. Hope M, Savva N, Whitehouse S, et al. Is it necessary to re-fuse a non-union of a Hallux metatarsophalangeal joint arthrodesis? Foot Ankle Int 2010;31(8):662–9.

20. Deorio JK. Technique tip: arthrodesis of the first metatarsophalangeal joint. Prevention of Excessive Dorsiflexion Foot and Ankle International 2007;28(6):746–7.

21. Bei C, Gross CE, Adams S, et al. Dual plating with bone block arthrodesis of the first metatarsophalangeal joint: a clinical retrospective review. Foot Ankle Surg 2015;21(4):235–9.

22. Buda M, Hagemeijer NC, Kink S, et al. Effect of fixation type and bone graft on tarsometatarsal fusion. Foot Ankle Int 2018;39(12):1394–402.

23. Coughlin MJ, Saltzman CL, Nunley JA 2nd. Angular measurements in the evaluation of hallux valgus deformities: a report of the ad hoc committee of the American Orthopaedic Foot & Ankle Society on angular measurements. Foot Ankle Int 2002;23(1):68–74.

24. Paley D, Herzenberg JE, Tetsworth K, et al. Deformity planning for frontal and sagittal plane corrective osteotomies. Orthop Clin North Am 1994;25(3):425–65.

25. Mashima N, Yamamoto H, Tsuboi I, et al. Correction of hallux valgus deformity using the center of rotation of angulation method. J Orthop Sci 2009;14(4):377–84.

26. Hunt KJ, Anderson RB. Biplanar proximal phalanx closing wedge osteotomy for hallux rigidus. Foot Ankle Int 2012;33(12):1043–50.

27. Cullen NP, Angel J, Singh D, et al. Clinical tip: revision first metatarsophalangeal joint arthrodesis for sagittal plane malunion with an opening wedge osteotomy using a small fragment block plate. Foot Ankle Int 2005;26(11):1001–3.

28. Attia AK, Mahmoud K, ElSweify K, et al. Donor site morbidity of calcaneal, distal tibial, and proximal tibial cancellous bone autografts in foot and ankle surgery. a systematic review and meta-analysis of 2296 bone grafts. Foot Ankle Surg 2022; 28(6):680–90.

29. Dimitriou R, Mataliotakis GI, Angoules AG, et al. Complications following autologous bone graft harvesting from the iliac crest and using the RIA: a systematic review. Injury 2011;42:S3–15.

30. Law RW, Langan TM, Consul DW, et al. Safety profile associated with calcaneal autograft harvesting using a reaming graft harvester. Foot Ankle Int 2020; 41(12):1487–92.

31. Garras DN, Durinka JB, Bercik M, et al. Conversion arthrodesis for failed first metatarsophalangeal joint hemiarthroplasty. Foot Ankle Int 2013;34(9):1227–32.

32. Luk PC, Johnson JE, McCormick JJ, et al. First metatarsophalangeal joint arthrodesis technique with interposition allograft bone block. Foot Ankle Int 2015;36(8): 936–43.

33. Burke JE, Shi GG, Wilke BK, et al. Allograft interposition bone graft for first metatarsal phalangeal arthrodesis: salvage after bone loss and shortening of the first ray. Foot Ankle Int 2021;42(8):969–75.

34. Lamm BM, Moore KR, Hentges M, et al. Avascular necrosis of the first metatarsal: a case of second metatarsal bone transport with external fixation. J Foot Ankle Surg 2021;60(3):595–9.

35. Liu F, Huang RK, Xie M, et al. Use of Masquelet's technique for treating the first metatarsophalangeal joint in cases of gout combined with a massive bone defect. Foot Ankle Surg 2018;24(2):159–63.

36. Abar B, Kwon N, Allen NB, et al. Outcomes of surgical reconstruction using custom 3d-printed porous titanium implants for critical-sized bone defects of the foot and ankle. Foot Ankle Int 2022;43(6):750–61.

37. Amin TH, Rathnayake V, Ramil M, et al. An innovative application of a computer aided design and manufacture implant for first metatarsal phalangeal joint arthrodesis: a case report. J Foot Ankle Surg 2020;59(6):1287–93.

38. Coriaty N, Pettibone K, Todd N, et al. Titanium scaffolding: an innovative modality for salvage of failed first ray procedures. J Foot Ankle Surg 2018;57(3):593–9.

39. Hollawell S, Coleman M. First metatarsophalangeal joint arthrodesis with titanium cage implant to address iatrogenic deformities of the first ray. Foot Ankle Surg, Techniques, Reports, & Cases 2022;2(2).

The Posttraumatic Tarsometatarsal Joints

Lant Abernathy, DPM, AACFAS*, Steven A. Tocci, DPM, AACFAS, Ryan T. Scott, DPM, FACFAS

KEYWORDS

- Midfoot fusion • Osteoarthritis • Tarsometatarsal • Midfoot arthrodesis

KEY POINTS

- Thorough clinical examination with a history of subtle or frank traumatic incident is key to correct diagnosis.
- After failure of conservative treatment modalities such as shoe modifications and corticosteroid injections, arthrodesis of the affected joints is typically necessary.
- Appropriate incision placement is key for adequate exposure of each tarsometatarsal joint for adequate joint preparation. It is also important to ensure a proper skin bridge when utilizing a multiple incision approach.
- Resection and curettage are techniques that can be used for joint preparation, although in situ curettage cannot correct for deformity.
- Compression bridge plating, interfragmentary screws, and nitinol staples are all options that have shown to achieve appropriate union rates.

INTRODUCTION

Midfoot arthritis, specifically of the tarsometatarsal joints (TMTJs), can cause significant pain and impairment of daily activities. The adult population can experience anywhere between 12% and 16% of symptomatic midfoot arthritis.[1] Several causes of TMTJ arthritis exist including Charcot neuroarthropathy, inflammatory disease, primary osteoarthritis, and most commonly posttraumatic osteoarthritis. It is estimated that up to 67% of TMTJ injuries are due to direct injuries such as motor vehicle accidents, falls from a height and direct crush injuries,[2] leaving approximately 33% resulting from low-energy trauma.[3] There is much controversy surrounding acute operative treatment of TMTJ injuries between open reduction and internal fixation versus primary arthrodesis. Regardless, the incidence of arthritis following TMTJ injuries is reported to be upward of 58%.[4] Thus, this article will focus primarily on the management and operative treatment strategies for painful posttraumatic TMTJ arthritis.

Financial Disclosures: RTS: Stryker.
The CORE Institute Advanced Foot and Ankle Reconstruction Fellowship, The CORE Institute, 9321 W Thomas Road Suite 205, Phoenix, AZ 85037, USA
* Corresponding author.
E-mail address: lant.abernathy54@gmail.com

Clin Podiatr Med Surg 40 (2023) 581–592
https://doi.org/10.1016/j.cpm.2023.05.003
0891-8422/23/© 2023 Elsevier Inc. All rights reserved.

ANATOMICAL AND BIOMECHANICAL REVIEW

The TMTJ, or Lisfranc joint, is an anatomically complex structure composed of the medial, central, and lateral columns. These columns are the articulation points of the more proximal tarsal bones, the 3 cuneiforms and cuboid, and the first through fifth metatarsals. The medial column is composed of the first metatarsal-medial cuneiform joint, which is a reniform or kidney-shaped joint. The central column is composed of the second TMTJ as well as the third TMTJ. The second TMTJ is described as a "keystone" joint that is recessed proximally compared with the other TMTJ joints. This geometric pattern adds to the strength of the arch and midfoot.[5] The Lisfranc ligament is an interosseous ligament that connects the medial cuneiform to the second metatarsal and is a commonly injured ligament in isolated injuries as well as fracture dislocations. The lateral column is composed of the fourth and fifth TMT joints, which is the articulation of the fourth and fifth metatarsals and the cuboid. These configurations of joints contribute to the transverse arch formation of the foot and are described as a "Roman arch." The cuneiforms and respective metatarsals are wedge shaped with the apex being plantarly, which adds innate stability to the arch. Strong interosseous as well as plantar ligaments support these joints on the tension side, whereas weaker dorsal ligaments are usually disrupted in fracture/dislocation injuries, which correlate to more commonly seen dorsal dislocation of the metatarsals.[5]

Biomechanically, the 3 columns of the Lisfranc joint vary in function as well as triplanar motion. Ouzounian and Shereff[6] described the motion of the columns individually, with the lateral column displaying the most motion followed by the medial, and the central column being the most rigid. The medial column is a critical part of first ray motion, with axes that function in a larger part to forefoot supination/pronation and is interconnected proximally to the chopart, subtalar, and ankle joints. The tibialis anterior and peroneus longus have antagonistic pull at their insertions on the plantar aspect of the medial column and can contribute to frontal plane rotation about the first ray. The lateral column has the peroneus brevis insertion at the fifth TMT joint that acts as a vital evertor of the foot. The midfoot is responsible for transferring load from the hindfoot to the forefoot. When the foot is supinated during toe-off, the transverse tarsal joints are locked allowing transfer of this load.[5]

CLINICAL EVALUATION

Patient history and clinical examination are key to an accurate diagnosis. Patients will often recall an inciting traumatic event in which they may or may not have sought treatment. Regardless, it has been estimated that approximately 20% of midfoot injuries are missed on initial examination.[7,8] The patient will often have complaints of aching or burning pain throughout the midfoot, especially with activity. The clinician can better localize which joints are affected by using the piano key test.[9] This is done by securing the midfoot and mobilizing individual metatarsal heads and examining for pain at the corresponding TMTJ. Physical examination will also often reveal palpable dorsal spurring along single or multiple TMTJs in a chronic presentation. Depending on the location and size of dorsal osteophytes, there can also be complaints of neuritis along the superficial cutaneous nerves of the dorsal foot, specifically with different types of shoe gear.

IMAGING

Imaging studies are also necessary for diagnosis and management. Standard weight-bearing anteroposterior (AP), oblique, and lateral radiographs will reveal joint space narrowing, sclerosis, and osteophytes at the arthritic joints and presence of any gross deformity. Gapping between the first and second metatarsals or second metatarsal-intermediate cuneiform step-off can also be seen on AP radiographs. In the case of previous trauma and continued pain, computed tomography (CT) scans can be helpful in assessing fracture healing, extent of arthritis, and degree of any subsequent deformity throughout the midfoot. Weight-bearing CT scans have become helpful in operative planning as well as in determining the standing architecture in the midfoot and any deformity that may need to be addressed simultaneously. If the patient is able to bear weight, a weight-bearing CT is recommended. MRI can also be a diagnostic modality similar to that of CT and will exhibit the amount and degree of arthritis within the individual TMTJs, as well as show bony edema and early developing arthritis of individual joints. These advanced imaging modalities can assist the surgeon in preoperative planning (**Figs. 1** and **2**).

CONSERVATIVE TREATMENT

Nonoperative treatment is typically used in the initial management and includes shoe gear modifications, orthotic inserts, full-length carbon fiber inserts, specific University of California-Berkley Labratory (UCBL) brace to limit midfoot motion, topical or oral anti-inflammatories, intra-articular corticosteroid injections, or a combination of treatments. Intra-articular injections can be both diagnostic and therapeutic. They can also better localize which joints are painful and can somewhat predict future success with arthrodesis. These injections can also determine if the pain is intra-articular or a result of dorsal osteophytes causing irritation and can drastically change surgical procedure. Protheroe and colleagues[10] looked at the efficacy of guided intra-articular injections for midfoot arthritis. They found that the self-reported foot and ankle score was significantly improved with an average duration of 4.5 months, with continued improvement from baseline at 12-month follow-up. They also found that patients with body mass index (BMI) greater than 30 had significantly lower improvement than those with BMI less than 30. If pain is unable to be managed with these options, surgical intervention is typically warranted. Khosla and colleagues[11] found in a cadaveric study that ultrasound (US)-guided needle injections were more accurate than direct palpation technique. US group found 10 of 14 of the first TMTJ and 8 of 14 of the second TMTJ while the direct palpation group found 3 of 14 of first TMTJ and 4 of 14 of second TMTJ (**Fig. 3**).

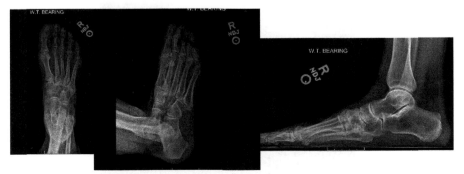

Fig. 1. Patient with chronic degenerative joint arthritis of the 2 to 3 tarsometatarsal and naviculo-cuneiform joints.

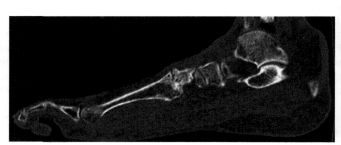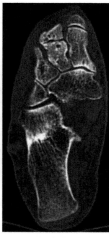

Fig. 2. Sagittal and coronal views of CT scan showing cystic changes and dorsal osteophytes secondary to TMT arthritis.

SURGICAL MANAGEMENT

Surgical management can be complicated, especially with multijoint disease. Outside of arthrodesis, there are limited reported surgical techniques available for those who may be poor arthrodesis candidates. Kindred and colleagues[12] performed deep peroneal neurectomy 5 cm proximal to the ankle joint on 26 patients with midfoot arthritis that either were not good surgical candidates or did not wish to adhere to postoperative protocol required for arthrodesis. They reported that 22/26 (85%) patients stated their expectations were met because of the neurectomy and that 76% would have the procedure done again. Of the 34 feet operated on, 9% did go on to require arthrodesis at an average of 40 months after their neurectomy. Gastrocnemius recession is another option with some reported positive outcomes, with the thought that decreasing the power of the gastrocsoleal complex can relieve plantigrade pressure

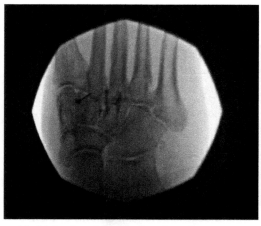

Fig. 3. Fluoroscopic-guided injections into the 2 to 3 TMTJs.

across the midfoot joints.[13] In this study, there was an average improvement of 44.63 points in midfoot American Orthopedi Foot and Ankle Society (AOFAS) score, with 7 of the 8 patients reporting complete resolution of symptoms. With an average follow-up of 28 months, all patients stated they were satisfied with their outcomes, and none of them went on to require midfoot arthrodesis by the end of the study.

Depending on symptoms, simple exostectomy of dorsal TMTJ spurs can alleviate irritation and pain in shoe gear. Typically, this gives relief to the dorsal neurovascular structures for a period. As stated above, it is critical to evaluate the source of pain clinically and intra-articular injections can add invaluable information. Patient expectations are also critical to understand and discuss in regards to the pathology and treatment goals.

Arthrodesis is often regarded as the gold standard treatment of posttraumatic TMT joints, more commonly performed on the medial and central columns. Several techniques as well as fixation constructs have been reported in the literature with varying outcomes and a lack of agreement.

Conventional fixation includes compression screws, locking or nonlocking plates, staples, or a combination of the above. Ettinger and colleagues[14] compared isolated 2 screw constructs versus screw and locking plate fixation for the medial and central columns. Screw and locking plate fixation demonstrated lower nonunion rates compared with isolated 1 or 2 screw fixation, or an isolated locking compression plate. Improvement in clinical and functional outcome scores, except for the University of California at Los Angeles scale. Dang and colleagues[1] described an isolated locking compression plate construct for longitudinal compression of the TMT joints and reported an 81.5% union rate among 62 patients at 7-year follow-up. Visual analog score (VAS) scores also decreased significantly from 5.9 preoperatively to 3.16 1 year postoperatively. They also found that increasing the number of joints fused per case increases the chance of nonunion. The average number of joints with successful fusion was 2.5 while the average number of joints leading to nonunion was 3.6. The first, second, and third TMTs had union rates of 83.8%, 91.5%, and 80.6%, respectively. Buda and colleagues[15] compared isolated plate fixation, 1 or 2 screw fixation, and hybrid fixation with nonunion rates of 16.4%, 5.8%, and 4.8%, respectively.

Dynamic staple fixation is also another construct that has some advantages compared with screws and plates. These include ease of insertion, decreased operating time, and a lower profile compared with plates. Some studies report approximately a 90% fusion rate while using staple fixation in the TMTJ as well as hindfoot joints.[16,17] Dock and colleagues[18] also described TMTJ arthrodesis using nitinol staples. Their study included 66 patients with statistically significant improved functional outcomes, including fusion rates of 89.7% with only 8 nonunions. Around 20% of patients had the staples removed secondary to hardware irritation compared with reported removal rate of 9% to 25% with conventional fixation.[19,20]

Lee and colleagues[21] retrospectively compared 4 different fixation constructs including a staple, single compression screw, compression screw and compression plate, and isolated compression plate. They reported that of the 95 patients in their study, the nonunion rates for the various constructs were 0%, 15.1%, 3.3%, and 15.8%, respectively.

Adjunctive use of bone graft can also aid in fusion rates, specifically with local defects and complicated comorbid patients. Autograft harvest techniques usually involve the ipsilateral iliac crest, proximal or distal tibia, and calcaneus. The donor site depends on the quantity required and skill set of the operating surgeon. Using autograft has more physiologic benefits of bone healing compared with allograft.

Donor site harvest can manifest complications such as fracture, pain, hematoma, neurovascular injury.[22,23] Allograft combined with adjunctive substitutes, such as bone marrow aspirate and platelet-derived growth factor, can be a safe alternative.[24] However, specifically in the foot and ankle, autogenous bone graft can be safely and efficiently harvested from the calcaneus.[23,25] Cancellous autograft can also be safely harvested from the medial aspect of the distal tibial metaphysis, which is also commonly used by the authors. Regardless of donor site, cancellous and structural autograft has shown to significantly decrease the rate of nonunion in foot and ankle fusions[15,26] (**Fig. 4**).

Various techniques for single and multiple TMTJ fusions have been described beyond a standard curettage technique. Johnson and Johnson[4] described a dowel arthrodesis technique in which an iliac crest autograft was harvested percutaneously and fixated in the arthrodesis site with 2 crossing k-wires. Out of 13 patients, 3 experienced nonunion and 11 experienced appropriate pain relief. Although this can be done in primary fusion, it is also an excellent option for revision TMTJ arthrodesis.[27] Traditional curettage or resection can cause iatrogenic shortening, which the trephine technique can help mitigate in revision surgeries. Reaming of the nonunion is achieved with the goal to maintain a 1 mm cortical edge medially and laterally, directions that add stability to the joint. Additionally, it is recommended that the plantar cortex not be violated. The matching diameter reamer is then used to remove a plug of cortico-cancellous graft from the calcaneus, which is then "press fit" into the nonunion site and fixated.

These techniques are less favorable when there is posttraumatic malunion or any other planar deformity, which demands correction. Presence of these deformities is usually corrected with saw resection to restore a more anatomic arch and metatarsal parabola. These can include sagittal and coronal plane deformities, hindfoot valgus, and forefoot abduction. Generally, deformity correction is needed when there is greater than 2 mm of displacement or 15° of angulation.[28] Identification of the apex of deformity is critical in correction. Radiographic parameters such as Meary's angle,

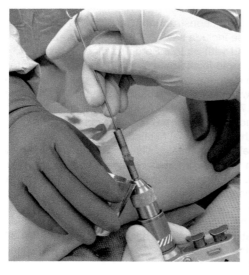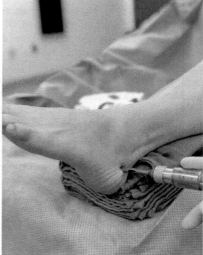

Fig. 4. Autograft harvest from the calcaneus with power trephine reamer.

medial wall alignment of the first metatarsal and medial cuneiform as well as the second metatarsal and middle cuneiform, and involvement of the lateral column with the fourth metatarsal aligned with the cuboid.[29] Use of structural allograft can be used to help correct length and alignment.[30] Concomitant soft tissue and bony procedures for pes planovalgus and pes cavus deformity associated with TMTJ arthritis are also performed.

Percutaneous techniques involving minimally invasive surgery have also been described. Lui described a technique as well as a case report involving arthroscopic-assisted TMTJ arthrodesis. A portal can be made for each TMTJ, using a 2.7-mm scope and shaver. The shaver is then used to denude all cartilage. Fixation included a single percutaneous screw for compression across each arthrodesis site. In this case series, arthrodesis of 1 to 3 TMTJ using arthroscopy achieved successful bony union and pain relief after an average of 20 weeks.[31]

Painful arthritis of the lateral column can be challenging to manage. Historically, arthrodesis has been avoided on the lateral column due to increased joint mobility and reportedly high nonunion rates. Because of this, interposition arthroplasty has more commonly been performed for the arthritic lateral column.

Shawen and colleagues[32] performed a retrospective case series on 13 patients who had fourth and fifth metatarsal-cuboid joint resection arthroplasties with spherical ceramic implants due to posttraumatic arthritis. At an average of 34 months follow-up, the mean AOFAS score was 53 points, which was an 87% improvement compared with preoperative scores. There was also a 42% improvement in VAS scores, and all 11 patients available for follow-up were satisfied with their outcome and would have the surgery again. There was only one complication, which was subsidence of the implant with no dislocations noted. Berlet and colleagues also had similar success with arthroplasty. They had 6 patients who completed their study with fourth and fifth metatarsal-cuboid joint resection with interposition using either peroneus tertius tendon or fourth toe extensor tendon rolled up in "anchovy" fashion and held in place with a percutaneous K wire. Seventy-five percent of those in the study reported satisfactory results. Interestingly, they found that those who had the most improvement in VAS scores after their diagnostic block had significantly better outcomes from the surgery.[33]

More recently, Derner and colleagues[34] described arthrodesis of the fourth and fifth TMT joints. The study population included patients with both Charcot neuroarthropathy and degenerative joint disease. Forty-five percent of the cohort in the degenerative joint disease group had an average of 16.3 weeks to radiographic union, statistically significant improvement in VAS scores, and an overall 10.8% nonunion rate between both groups.

Postsurgical complications can vary. These include but are not limited to wound healing problems/infection (3%), peripheral nerve injury (9%), nonunion (3%–8%), painful neuroma formation (7%), and screw irritation or breakage (9%).[1,5,14] Furthermore, adjacent joint arthritis (4.5%) is also a concern postarthrodesis because the midfoot, or an extent of it, is locked and more motion occurs at the proximal and distal joints of the foot as compensation.[20] Patient comorbidities, smoking, and BMI all have higher risks of complications.

AUTHORS' PREFERRED SURGICAL TECHNIQUES
Single-Incision Approach

During the single approach for an isolated or multi-TMTJ fusion of the second and third TMT, the incision is placed off the lateral aspect of the second metatarsal base (**Fig. 5**).

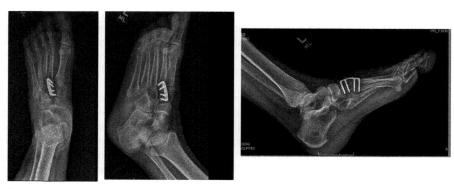

Fig. 5. Single-incision approach with staple fixation.

If a patient had previous ORIF with plates, then the previous incision site is used as our incision. Incision is deepened through the subcutaneous issue with care taken to identify and retract the neurovascular bundle. The neurovascular bundle should be located on the medial aspect of the surgical incision. The underlying muscle belly of the extensor hallucis brevis will then be encountered. This is typically retracted medially. Direct dissection down to the level of the TMTJ is then performed. In the case of previous ORIF, there will be a large amount of scar tissue present that will need to be dissected through carefully. The dorsal capsule is then sharply incised. We keep the intermetatarsal ligaments attached in between the second and third TMTJs. This way, when we distract one joint, the other will also distract as one unit and give us better visual aid into both joints. Hardware is removed at this point if present. We prefer a pin distractor in assistance for visualization and preparation for arthrodesis. The second and third TMTJs are then prepped with a series of curettes, osteotomes, and a rotary burr. The authors prefer using curettage and the use of a resurfacing burr for debridement of the remaining cartilage and subchondral plate. Curettage is preferred by us to prevent as much shortening as possible. If there is any planal deformity, the use of a sagittal saw to correct the deformity is used, although it does cause shortening. The subchondral bone is then penetrated with a drill bit and "fish scaled" with a curved osteotome. Bone graft is then placed into the arthrodesis site. The authors prefer autologous bone graft harvested from the calcaneus, a technique described by Law and colleagues.[23] A small 1-cm incision is made on the lateral posterior wall of the calcaneus. Care is taken to avoid the sural nerve and the peroneal tendons. Using a reamer, around 5 cc of bone graft is harvested. Depending on how many joints need fusion, approximately 1 to 2 cc is put in each joint. For neglected Lisfranc injuries in which there is a persistent diastasis between the second metatarsal base and medial cuneiform, it is necessary to recess the metatarsal proximally to restore the keystone aspect of the midfoot. Through this incision, the diastasis is debrided of scar tissue that would impede reduction. Spot welding of this area can be used with the above-mentioned burr. The lesser metatarsals are then reduced in all 3 planes and pinned in place. Fluoroscopic examination is then performed showing appropriate reduction of the lesser joints. Solid rigid fixation is then used via surgeon preference. Dynamic compression plates with eccentric drilling is the author's preferred fixation construct. If joint apposition is difficult manually, a point-to-point clamp can also be used to gain compression. Alternative fixation is warranted for limitations with small amounts of bone stock secondary to patients' anatomy or bone voids created from previous hardware. Moreover, if the patient's anatomy is too limited for a plate that may impinge proximally on the naviculo-cuneiform joint, staple fixation may be utilized.

Dual-Incision Approach

For a dual-incision approach for a multi-TMTJ fusion, we prefer a dorsal-medial based incision over the first TMTJ, as well as a secondary incision over the lateral aspect of the second metatarsal base (**Figs. 6** and **7**). It is necessary to have an appropriate skin bridge, preferably greater than 2 cm to avoid any wound complications. For the medial-based incision, the incision is deepened through the subcutaneous tissue with care taken to identify and retract all neurovascular structures. Branches of the saphenous vein and saphenous nerve will be in the direct line of visualization during this approach. Dissection should be taken carefully around the structures retracting the structures inferior. Dorsally, the extensor hallucis longus will be encountered. An incision directly down the level of bone should be made between the saphenous vein and the extensor hallucis longus. Preparation for arthrodesis is performed in a similar fashion as listed in the single joint fusion. Once again, we prefer to use the pin distractor for visualization and aid in preparation for arthrodesis. The distal pin is placed dorsally in the first metatarsal base. This will later be used as the counter sink and entry drill for the home run screw across the first TMTJ. The authors prefer an interfragmentary compression screw across the first TMTJ along with a medial neutralization plate. Care should be taken to place the medial plate in such a position to minimize irritation of the tibialis anterior tendon.

POSTOPERATIVE PROTOCOL

Patients will be non–weight-bearing in a posterior short leg splint for 2 weeks. At 2 weeks, patient sutures are removed if warranted and placed in a non–weight-bearing short leg cast for the next 4 to 6 weeks. At 6 to 8 weeks postoperatively, patients are taken out of a non–weight-bearing cast and placed in a tall pneumatic walking boot and are weight-bearing as tolerated for the next 4 weeks, granted that radiographs at this time show appropriate arthrodesis progression. At 10 to 12 weeks, postoperatively, patients transition into a stiff soled shoe with an over the counter stiff carbon fiber foot plate.

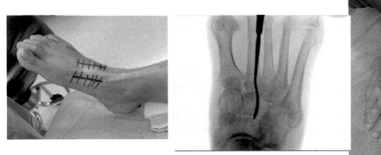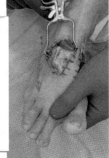

Fig. 6. Incision placement and dissection for the multi-TMTJ fusion.

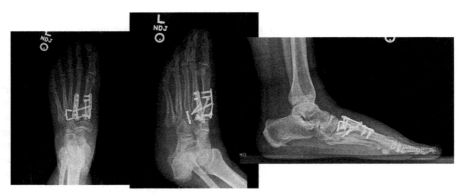

Fig. 7. Multi-TMTJ fusion with plate and staple construct.

SUMMARY

- Appropriate physical evaluation will increase the success rate of midfoot pathology
- Advanced imaging is critical in diagnosis and management of the arthritic midfoot
- Rigid fixation constructs with compression through the TMT joint increase in the success of arthrodesis
- Use of autograft has been shown to increase fusion rates in both primary and revision midfoot arthrodesis
- The authors typically use compression plating for the first and second TMT joints and use either a single compression screw or a nitinol staple for the third TMT

CLINICS CARE POINTS

- Appropriate physical evaluation will increase the success rate of midfoot pathology
- Advanced imaging is critical in diagnosis and management of the arthritic midfoot
- Rigid fixation constructs with compression through the TMT joint increase in the success of arthrodesis
- Use of autograft/allograft has shown to increase fusion rates in both primary and revision midfoot arthrodesis
- The authors typically use compression plating for the first and second TMT joints and use either a single compression screw or a nitinol staple for the third TMT

REFERENCES

1. Dang DY, Flint WW, Haytmanek CT, et al. Locked dorsal compression plate arthrodesis for degenerative arthritis of the midfoot. J Foot Ankle Surg 2020; 59(6):1171–6.
2. Myerson MS, Fisher RT, Burgess AR, et al. Fracture dislocations of the tarsometatarsal joints: end results correlated with pathology and treatment. Foot Ankle 1986;6(5):225–42.
3. Vuori JP, Aro HT. Lisfranc joint injuries: trauma mechanisms and associated injuries. J Trauma 1993 Jul;35(1):40–5.

4. Johnson JE, Johnson KA. Dowel arthrodesis for degenerative arthritis of the tarsometatarsal (Lisfranc) joints. Foot Ankle 1986;6(5):243–53.
5. Kurup H, Vasukutty N. Midfoot arthritis- current concepts review. J Clin Orthop Trauma 2020;11(3):399–405.
6. Ouzounian TJ, Shereff MJ. In vitro determination of midfoot motion. Foot Ankle 1989;10:140–6.
7. Marín-Peña OR, Recio FV, Gómez TS, et al. Fourteen years follow up after Lisfranc fracture-dislocation: functional and radiological results. Injury 2012;43:S79–82.
8. Sethuraman U, Grover SK, Kannikeswaran N. Tarsometatarsal injury in a child. Pediatr Emerg Care 2009;25:594–6.
9. Keiserman LS, Cassandra J, Amis JA. The piano key test: a clinical sign for the identification of subtle tarsometatarsal pathology. Foot Ankle Int 2003 May; 24(5):437–8.
10. Protheroe D, Gadgil A. Guided intra-articular corticosteroid injections in the midfoot. Foot Ankle Int 2018;39(8):1001–4.
11. Khosla S, Thiele R, Baumhauer JF. Ultrasound guidance for intra-articular injections of the foot and ankle. Foot Ankle Int 2009;30(9):886–90.
12. Kindred KB, Wavrunek MR, Blacklidge DK, et al. Deep peroneal neurectomy for midfoot arthritis. J Foot Ankle Surg 2021;60(2):276–82.
13. Anselmo DS, Thatcher L, Erfle D. Gastrocnemius recession as an alternative to midfoot arthrodesis for painful midfoot arthritis. J Foot Ankle Surg 2020;59(5): 1106–8.
14. Ettinger S, Altemeier A, Stukenborg-Colsman C, et al. Comparison of isolated screw to plate and screw fixation for tarsometatarsal arthrodesis including clinical outcome Predictors. Foot Ankle Int 2021;42(6):734–43.
15. Buda M, Hagemeijer NC, Kink S, et al. Effect of fixation type and bone graft on tarsometatarsal fusion. Foot Ankle Int 2018;39:1394–402.
16. Schipper ON, Ellington JK. Nitinol compression staples in foot and ankle surgery. Orthop Clin North Am 2019;50(3):391–9.
17. Schipper ON, Ford SE, Moody PW, et al. Radiographic results of nitinol compression staples for hindfoot and midfoot arthrodeses. Foot Ankle Int 2018;39(2): 172–9.
18. Dock CC, Freeman KL, Coetzee JC, et al. Outcomes of nitinol compression staples in tarsometatarsal fusion. Foot Ankle Orthop 2020;5(3). 2473011420944904.
19. Jung HG, Myerson MS, Schon LC. Spectrum of operative treatments and clinical outcomes for atraumatic osteoarthritis of the tarsometatarsal joints. Foot Ankle Int 2007;28(4):482–9.
20. Nemec SA, Habbu RA, Anderson JG, et al. Outcomes following midfoot arthrodesis for primary arthritis. Foot Ankle Int 2011;32(4):355–61.
21. Lee W, Prat D, Wapner KL, et al. Comparison of 4 different fixation strategies for midfoot arthrodesis: a retrospective Comparative study. Foot Ankle Spec 2021. https://doi.org/10.1177/19386400211032482. 19386400211032482.
22. Klifto C, Gandi S, Sapienza A. Bone graft options in upper-extremity surgery. J Hand Surg 2018;43(8):755–61.
23. Law RW, Langan TM, Consul DW, et al. Safety profile associated with calcaneal autograft harvesting using a reaming graft harvester. Foot Ankle Int 2020; 41(12):1487–92.
24. Scott RT, McAlister JE, Rigby RB. Allograft bone: what is the Role of platelet-derived growth factor in hindfoot and ankle fusions. Clin Podiatr Med Surg 2018;35(1):37–52.

25. Roukis T. A simple technique for harvesting autogenous bone grafts from the calcaneus. Foot Ankle Int 2006;27(11):998–9.
26. DiGiovanni CW, Lin SS, Daniels TR, et al. The importance of Sufficient graft material in achieving foot or ankle fusion. J Bone Joint Surg Am 2016;98(15):1260–7.
27. Grambart ST, Reese ER. Trephine procedure for revision tarsometatarsal arthrodesis nonunion. Clin Podiatr Med Surg 2020;37(3):447–61.
28. Komenda GA, Myerson MS, Biddinger KR. Results of arthrodesis of the tarsometatarsal joints after traumatic injury. J Bone Joint Surg Am 1996;78:1665–76.
29. Zonno AJ, Myerson MS. Surgical correction of midfoot arthritis with and without deformity. Foot Ankle Clin 2011;16(1):35–47.
30. Myerson MS, Neufeld SK, Uribe J. Fresh-frozen structural allografts in the foot and ankle. J Bone Joint Surg Am 2005;87:113–20.
31. Lui TH. Arthroscopic tarsometatarsal arthrodesis. Arthrosc Tech 2016;5(6): e1311–6.
32. Shawen SB, Anderson RB, Cohen BE, et al. Spherical ceramic interpositional arthroplasty for basal fourth and fifth metatarsal arthritis. Foot Ankle Int 2007;28(8): 896–901.
33. Berlet GC, Hodges Davis W, Anderson RB. Tendon arthroplasty for basal fourth and fifth metatarsal arthritis. Foot Ankle Int 2002;23(5):440–6.
34. Derner R, Derner BS, Olsen A. Fusion of the tarsometatarsal joints: a focus on lateral column fusion nonunion rates. J Foot Ankle Surg 2020;59(4):704–10.

Management of Midfoot Charcot

Minimally Invasive Techniques and Improved Fixation

Sara Mateen, DPM, AACFAS[a], Kwasi Y. Kwaadu, DPM, FACFAS[b,c,d,*]

KEYWORDS

- Charcot neuroarthropathy • Midfoot charcot • Internal fixation
- Intramedullary beaming • Surgical techniques • Minimally invasive surgery

KEY POINTS

- Understand the etiology of Charcot neuroarthropathy and how it affects osseous architecture.
- Discuss new minimally invasive surgical concepts of Charcot neuroarthropathy reconstructive surgery to decrease soft tissue insult with the hope of decreasing wound healing complications and increase overall success rates.
- Discuss a newer take on reconstructive surgery.

INTRODUCTION

Charcot neuroarthropathy (CNA) was originally described by William Musgrave in 1703 as a result of venereal disease. However, Jean-Martin Charcot later made the connection to neuropathies associated with spinal cord injuries secondary to Tabes dorsalis.[1] While alcoholic neuropathy, spinal cord injuries, syphilis, and syringomyelia remained etiologies for CNA, Diabetes Mellitus gained an association in the 1930's and remains the most common predisposing etiology.[2] In Charcot neuropathy, peripheral neuropathy with loss of sensation will precede any sort of complications to the foot and ankle joints. This neuropathy may be caused by hyperglycemia, oxidative stress, adipose toxicity, polyol pathway, elevated inflammatory markers, and overall accumulation of advanced glycation end products.[3–12]

^a Foot and Ankle Deformity and Orthoplastics, Rubin Institute for Advanced Orthopedics, 2401 West Belvedere Avenue, Baltimore, MD 21215, USA; ^b Department of Podiatric Surgery, Temple University School f Podiatric Medicine, 148 North 8th Street, Philadelphia, PA, USA; ^c Podiatric Surgical Residency, Temple University School f Podiatric Medicine, 148 North 8th Street, Philadelphia, PA, USA; ^d Department of Surgery, Temple University School f Podiatric Medicine, 148 North 8th Street, Philadelphia, PA, USA
* Corresponding author. 148 N 8th Street, Philadelphia, PA 19107.
E-mail address: kwasi.kwaadu@temple.edu

Clin Podiatr Med Surg 40 (2023) 593–611
https://doi.org/10.1016/j.cpm.2023.05.004
0891-8422/23/© 2023 Elsevier Inc. All rights reserved.

podiatric.theclinics.com

The pathophysiology of CNA has been associated with three reported theories: neurotraumatic, neurovascular, and neurohumoral theory. In the neurotraumatic theory, the eponymous German researcher, Jean-Martin Charcot hypothesized that significant sensory deficits in the neuropathic patient lead to lost pain perception. This loss coupled with repetitive minor trauma or injury to the foot lead to microfracture, microdislocations, and further progression of the deformity. This subsequently led to increased pressures on the surrounding soft tissue, ulcerations, infection, and amputation.[13–15] The neurovascular theory hypothesized that autonomic neuropathy impaired the vascular reflexes of the arteriovenous (AV) shunting causing increased arterial perfusion. Increased blood flow leads to increased bone resorption and reduced bone mineral density, predisposing patients for collapse and fragmentation.[16–21] Despite reports of increased perfusion and bounding pedal pulses, diabetics have a higher prevalence of peripheral vascular disease with calcification in smooth muscle of arterial walls.[21,22] Recent literature has suggested a combination of the traumatic and vascular theories play a role in the development of Charcot neuroarthropathy resulting in a significant mechanical and structural breakdown of the foot and ankle.[22]

Another studied theory is the neurohumoral theory, hypothesizing that sensory and sympathetic nerves affect the Charcot joints and subsequently, alter the inflammatory process. A study performed by Koeck and colleagues evaluated the density of sympathetic and sensory substance P-positive (SP+) nerve fibers in Charcot joints and compared this to osteoarthritic joints.[23] There was a marked loss of sympathetic nerve fibers in the chronically inflamed tarsus joint. However, the overall density of sympathetic nerve fibers in skin, synovial tissue, and bone, was lower in Charcot joints.

Pathophysiology

CNA is presently believed as an osteoclast-osteoblast imbalance with an uncontrolled inflammatory cascade of proinflammatory cytokines such as interleukin (IL)-1.[24] This results in an increased osteoclastic state, fracture, which further potentiates an inflammatory process through the receptor activation of nuclear factor kappa-B ligand (RANK-L) pathway. The influence of the RANK-L pathway has been identified in inflammatory imbalances in osteoporosis, inflammatory arthritides, and osteogenic malignancy.[25]

It is important to recognize early signs of CNA as continued fragmentation can lead to collapse. As the disease progresses, there will be increased loosening, fragmentation, and breakdown of joints and osseous structures. Early clinical symptoms may include edema, erythema, and warmth with joint effusion in the absence of radiographic.[24–26] Shibata and colleagues added a stage 0 to the established Eichenholtz classification which describes an inflammatory foot without the radiographic changes as seen in stage I.[27] As CNA progresses to stage I, clinical symptoms resemble those of stage 0 but with radiographic evidence of fragmentation, intra-articular loose bodies, subchondral osteopenia, and ligamentous laxity.[24–26] Stage II defines the coalescence phase in which there is radiographic evidence of debris, sclerosis, and fusion of larger osseous fragments. Clinically, there is decreased warmth, swelling, and erythema.[24–26] Finally, stage III represents the reconstructive stage with radiographic evidence of rounding and smoothing of bone fragments, along with fibrous ankyloses.[24–26] In stage III, there is little clinical edema, warmth, or erythema. The most common location for Charcot breakdown is the tarsometatarsal joint, which can lead to rocker bottom deformity with plantar, medial, or lateral osseous prominences with or without valgus deformity of the forefoot. There are opposing forces from the ankle extensors and a contracted Achilles tendon, exacerbating the dislocation of the midfoot or "bayonetting" of the forefoot on the hindfoot. This typically follows a dorsolateral pattern due to the longitudinal pull of the anterior and posterior compartment muscle groups.[24–26]

Managing Midfoot Charcot Neuroarthropathy

One of the most difficult challenges is differentiating osteomyelitis from CNA as these can occur simultaneously, particularly in the presence of a current or prior ulceration.[28] The incidence of diabetic foot ulcerations is approximately 15%, with the rate increasing to 37% in those with diabetic CNA[29–31] (**Fig. 1**). In the presence of osteomyelitis with ulceration, infection will need to be addressed and Charcot reconstructive surgery secondarily delayed until infection is either irradicated or successfully treated with serial debridements and intravenous antibiotics. In this respect, a staged approached should be considered for infection management with serial debridements, microbiology, and pathologic investigation, and ultimately stabilization of the foot and ankle through external fixation. Once the infection is appropriately managed, definitive reconstruction can proceed through either internal fixation, external fixation, or a combination of both. Radiographs and commuted tomography (CT) scanning may be useful in detecting early stages of disease, as plain radiography has low sensitivity and specificity (<50%).[29–31] Magnetic resonance imaging (MRI) may be a useful imaging modality in detecting early changes of Charcot and abscesses, but may lack the ability to differentiate osteomyelitis and Charcot arthropathy.[32] Bone biopsy and cultures remain the gold standard in diagnosing osteomyelitis and should be utilized when there is clinical suspicion of underlying infection.

The vascular status is of vital importance as in the absence thereof, salvage is moot.[33] Oxygenation and cellular nutrients are vital for healing and can only be

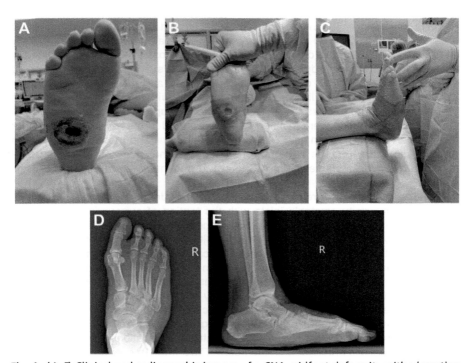

Fig. 1. (A–E) Clinical and radiographic images of a CNA midfoot deformity with ulceration.

delivered by a patent arterial inflow.[34] This is also equally important when considering local or free flaps for large Charcot wound defects followed by extensive debridement. A detailed vascular examination is imperative. This includes clinical pulse examination, skin color and pedal hair evaluation, assessing dermal atrophy, and temperature of the skin. A Doppler can provide additional information and determine sufficient or insufficient blood flow to the targeted area.[35,36] Angiography, arterial duplex ultrasound, ankle brachial index (ABI), pulse volume recordings (PVRs) will provide the necessary layer of information of vascular supply.[35,36] Vascular consultation is necessary if arterial perfusion is limited.

The ultimate goal of Charcot neuroarthropathy is to achieve a plantigrade and braceable foot. Charcot Restraint Orthotic Walking (CROW) boots are beneficial within the first 6 months to a year following successful reconstruction, but for many patients, can make ambulation arduous and really should be considered when the absence thereof would create catastrophic disaster and failure.[37] In the absence of infection or ulcerations, rocker bottom soled shoes with a rigid shank are recommended. Ankle foot orthosis (AFO) with custom shoes can also be used for the conservative management of some milder Charcot deformities without marked instability. In the non-plantigrade foot with or without ulcerations, surgical intervention is indicated, either in the form of wound debridement, exostectomy, and/or deformity correction with the use of internal and/or external fixation.

New Surgical Considerations in Managing Charcot Neuroarthropathy

Early recognition and treatment are essential in CNA for limb preservation. One of the major goals of surgery is to achieve an infection-free plantigrade foot that could be maintained with long-term therapeutic footwear. From a health care perspective, patients with CNA contribute to higher costs and are at an eight times greater risk of major lower extremity amputation. The initial cost of Charcot reconstruction can exceed USD 55,000 and can be substantially greater if revisional surgery is warranted.[37] Albright and colleagues examined the cost-effectiveness (defined by lifetime costs, quality-adjusted life-years [QUALYs], and incremental cost-effectiveness ratio [ICER] of surgical reconstruction and its alternatives [primary transtibial amputation and lifetime bracing) for adults with unstable midfoot Charcot and diabetes.[37] The authors discovered that the high upfront costs associated with surgical reconstruction were justified when performed in the early stages of Charcot neuroarthropathy, such as those without ulcerations and those without uncomplicated ulcerations.[37] The authors concluded that the data collected supported reconstruction for unstable midfoot Charcot in patients with an intact soft tissue envelope.[37]

Previous indications for reconstructive surgery include an unbraceable foot, limb-threatening deformity, unstable joints with the tenting of surrounding soft tissues, and recalcitrant ulcerations with or without concomitant osteomyelitis.[37–45] Patients with CNA have reduced functional ability, vitality, and social functioning compared to patients with diabetes alone. While these indications still hold true and are still major considerations, reconstruction prior to ulceration or catastrophic collapse has demonstrated good short-term results.[37–45] Newer considerations for reconstructive surgery include an unstable midfoot Charcot deformity with an intact soft tissue envelope, Meary's angle less than 27°, even without a rocker bottom deformity. As the clinical picture declines and patients develop worsening infection, there is ultimately a higher cost of reconstruction, higher rate of post-operative complications, and shorter life expectancies with less predictable outcomes.[37] Thus, it is our opinion that addressing midfoot Charcot before major complications arise may serve the patient's best interest and serve the health care community at large by potentially reducing hospital costs related to more complicated reconstruction.

Minimally Invasive Surgical Techniques for Midfoot Charcot Neuroarthropathy

Minimally invasive surgery has regained popularity in recent years particularly as it pertains to bunion surgery.[46–51] Bosch and colleagues provided some of the earliest publications on minimally invasive hallux valgus correction utilizing a less than 1 cm incision over the first metatarsal head and neck. Their technique involving fixation with a 2-mm Steinmann pin resulted in excellent radiographic outcomes and patient satisfaction up to 81% with 95% patient satisfaction at the long-term follow-up.[47,48] Giannini and Isham corroborated these outcomes with similar findings and concluded success with minimally invasive hallux valgus correction.[49,50] Recent publications by Siddiqui and colleagues have also reported success with minimally invasive hallux valgus surgery with over 300 procedures performed.[46] In North America, minimally invasive surgery was introduced in the 1980's but due to inexperience and inefficient technology, the results were suboptimal and these techniques faded out of favor. With improved techniques and technology, recent outcomes have proved more favorable.

With more familiarity, surgeon creativity with minimally invasive techniques are extending applications. Beyond hallux valgus reconstruction, these concepts of minimally invasive surgery are gaining popularity in hammertoe correction, exostectomies, calcaneal osteotomies, and recently with CNA reconstruction. Principles of deformity correction in this case are applied with minimal incision or percutaneous techniques. With this, surgeons ensure minimal soft-tissue disruption, preserve vascularity, obtain anatomic reduction when reasonably achievable in order to improve mechanical realignment, maintain relative stability of osteotomies or arthrodesis sites, and encourage early mobilization when indicated.[46] These principles have been adapted in Charcot reconstructive surgery, specifically with intramedullary column beaming. Advocacy of these techniques has led to the given acronym NEMISIS: neuropathic minimally invasive surgery.[51] It is an important concept in CNA as patients are already at increased risk of wound complications, hardware failure, and post-operative infection. With minimally invasive techniques, there is minimal disruption of the soft tissue envelope, osteotomies are performed with 20-mm long side-cutting burrs (2-3 mm in diameter) with or without pre-placed 2-mm Kirschner guide wires. The morselized bone paste bone is squeezed out and irrigated before intramedullary beams are delivered.[51]

Lamm and colleagues coined the term intramedullary foot fixation (IMFF) which has various advantages with midfoot Charcot neuroarthropathy reconstructive surgery which include minimally invasive surgical techniques, adjacent joint fixation, stable intraosseous fixation, anatomic realignment, preservation of foot length, and also if needed, combination of external fixation.[44] These authors concluded that IMFF advocated for adjacent fusion beyond the level of Charcot collapse by providing stability and dispersing the axial load while healing occurred[44,52] Another advantage to IMFF is that it provides rigid intimately-fitted intramedullary/intraosseous fixation both in width and length similar to intramedullary nail fixation in axial long bone fractures. This fixation technique is ideal in Charcot reconstructive surgery because Charcot bone is weaker than normal bone and placement of IMFF avoided added cortical bone stress and provides greater stability for each osseous segment.[53]

Reconstruction of the Midfoot in Charcot Neuroarthropathy

CNA's primary effects at the tarsometatarsal and naviculocuneiform joints are influenced by the cantilever bending forces in the midfoot.[38,45] This can be further impaired with continued weight-bearing and as a result, the anterior calcaneus plantarflexes increasing midfoot pressures and risk ulceration.[38,45] A tight posterior muscle group can exacerbate these pressures of osseous, ligamentous, and tendinous structures further exacerbating midfoot breakdown. The deforming force of the Achilles tendon can be further exacerbated with a combination of joint immobilization and non-enzymatic glycation and is relieved by lengthening the tendon via the Hoke triple hemi-section.[38,45]

With minimally invasive techniques, the concepts of proper joint preparation to facilitate fusion still hold true.[45] Proper joint preparation can be performed with smaller incisions and safe power burrs that are high torque and low speed to reduce the risk of thermal necrosis. Fenestration of the subchondral plate also can be performed through these smaller incisions to expose more of the underlying cancellous bone to increase osseous perfusion in order to facilitate consolidation.

Superconstructs have guided surgeons in major Charcot reconstruction success. Based on the current IMFF guidelines, surgeons are recommended to (1) extending the arthrodesis far beyond the zone of injury to maximize contact between the fixation and solid bone that has not been compromised by the disease process (2) resection of underlying bone to shorten the osseous architecture to allow a strong reconstruction without soft tissue tension (3) utilization of strong fixation without compromising surrounding periosteum (4) fixation devices placed in biomechanical optimal locations such as intramedullary bolts.[45]

Solid intramedullary bolts and cannulated beams can be delivered through small incisions to limit soft tissue dissection. The bolts are mechanically optimal because they resist cantilever bending forces that could gap the plantar aspect of the reconstruction, further increasing the risk of dorsal malunion.[45,51–53] Pre-operatively, the width of the metatarsal canal is measured to ensure a proper sized bolt. Current medial column intramedullary bolts range from 6.5mm to 8 mm. 5 mm diameter bolts are commonly used for the lesser metatarsals, delivered through the MTPJs. The medial column intramedullary bolt can be supplemented with a blocking screw distally to limit micromotion and decrease the risk of hardware failure and/or non-union.[45,51–53] To accommodate the transversely oriented blocking screw, the intramedullary bolt is advanced further beyond the metatarsal head (**Fig. 2**). The lateral column bolts gain proximal hold through the calcaneus and can be inserted in a retrograde or antegrade fashion. Sammarco and colleagues in a series of 22 patients using beams alone had higher union rates compared to previous studies with 16 osseous unions at 6 months and all patients returned to independent ambulation at 10 months.[45,53]

TECHNIQUE
Posterior Muscle Group Lengthening

The procedure generally begins with posterior muscular group lengthening. While the gastrocnemius recession reduces the risk of overlengthening and calcaneal gait, patients with midfoot Charcot present with significant posterior muscular and capsular contractures that are not adequately released with the gastrocnemius recession. Consequently, it is the author's recommendation that this patient population benefit from formal tendoachilles lengthening. The Hoke triple hemisection tendoachilles lengthening significantly attenuates the plantarflexory deforming cantilever midfoot forces imparted by the combination of the hindfoot equinus contracture and ground reactive forces (**Fig. 3**). Tendoachilles lengthening is recommended as a gastrocnemius recession will under correct the hindfoot equinus and increased the risk of recurrence.[45] This effectively creates an apropulsive gait, further diffusing the deforming

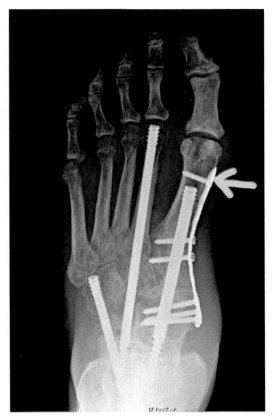

Fig. 2. Radiographic image demonstrating the blocking screw pointed out by the blue arrow

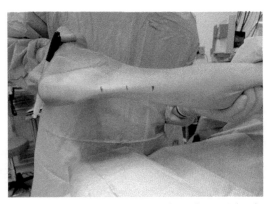

Fig. 3. Dermatologic marking in preparation for the triple hemisection Achilles lengthening.

forces. As part of the correction, dorsiflexing the unstable midfoot reduces the corrective effect of the procedure. Instead of dorsiflexing the unstable midfoot, the author instead recommends inserting a percutaneous 5 mm Schanz pin from the posterior calcaneus and using that instead to simulate the Essex-Lopresti maneuver, plantarflexing the posterior calcaneus in order to perform the muscular lengthening (**Fig. 4**). This is important as dorsiflexion of the forefoot may lead to the movement arm being concentrated at the unstable midfoot, leading to insufficient hindfoot correction. Once complete, two 0.062-inch Kirschner wires, or two 2 mm Steinman pins are used to percutaneously transfixate the tibiotalar articulation (**Fig. 5**). At this point, the forefoot

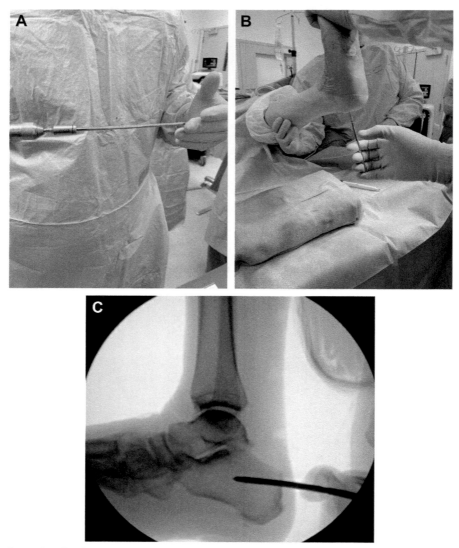

Fig. 4. (A–C) Schanz pin placed in the calcaneus used to facilitate Achilles lengthening following the triple hemisection.

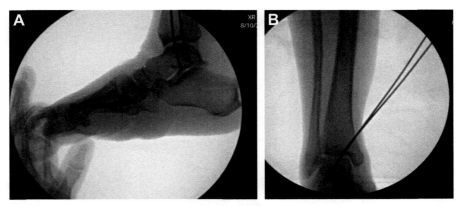

Fig. 5. (*A* and *B*) Transfixation of the tibiotalar articulation to maintain the equinal correction.

and midfoot deformities are then reconstructed toward the proximal reference, the hindfoot.

Joint Preparation

Attention is then directed toward the coalesced tarsometatarsal joints. Under fluoroscopic guidance, a small incision is made at the medial aspect of the joint, at the midpoint of its sagittal height, in order to facilitate effective preparation of the entire height of the joint, avoiding over resection of either the dorsal or plantar aspect of the joint. A hemostat is used to dissect down to the bone. The burr is then inserted and used to morselize the joint and approximately 2 mm on either side of the joint to confirm exposure of raw cancellous bone. In addition to the exposure of the raw bone, this will result in desirable inherent shortening of the underlying osseous architecture which effectively offloads the soft tissues even further (**Fig. 6**). While aggressive in bone, the burr is forgiving to the surrounding soft tissue because the surgeon has to lean the burr into the target tissue to facilitate resection. With patience and under fluoroscopic guidance, depending on the width of the foot and the length of the burr, the first through fourth tarsometatarsal joints can be prepped from a single 0.5-1 cm medial incision. If needed, a separate lateral incision of similar size can be made along the lateral fourth tarsometatarsal joint. Attention can then be directed toward the medial naviculocuneiform joint, which can be prepped in a similar fashion to the tarsometatarsal joints as these joints are similarly planar in their morphology. As this joint complex does not extend beyond the lateral boundary of the third metatarsal, it can generally be prepped effectively through a single medial incision. Nevertheless, when needed, a lateral incision can be performed to facilitate preparation (**Fig. 7**). The talonavicular joint preparation generally requires medial and lateral percutaneous incisions due to the concavity of the acetabular pedis (**Fig. 8**). The subtalar joint is difficult to access percutaneously with the instrumentation through the medial approach, so a separate lateral portal is recommended. The calcaneocuboid joint is accessed with fluoroscopic assistance through a lateral percutaneous incision. Long handheld curettes and joint preparatory instruments can be used to further evacuate the morselized bone and cartilage (**Fig. 9**). The sites are irrigated in traditional fashion with bulb syringes but smaller portals can be irrigated with the assistance of a 20 cc syringe with a 16-gauge angiocath needle.

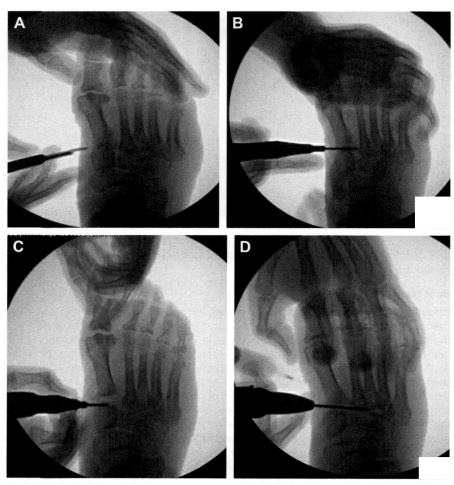

Fig. 6. (*A–D*) Fluoroscopy demonstrating percutaneous incisions placed and minimally invasive burr demonstrating tarsometatarsal joint preparations.

Reduction and Fixation

Consistent with the superconstuct guidelines of resecting bone in order to functionally lengthen the underlying soft tissues, bone grafting is generally not recommended. And in the spirit of minimally invasive techniques, plate fixation is not recommended. Therefore, preoperative measurements of the inner metatarsal canals can help provide the surgeon an idea of the desired intramedullary screw diameters. In preparation for fixation, the first metatarsal head is accessed by a dorsal metatarsophalangeal joint (MTPJ) incision (**Fig. 10**). Depending on the motion available at the joint, the metatarsal head can also be accessed plantarly, but requires more dissection, with care taken not to damage the long flexor tendon. The guide wire is introduced under fluoroscopic guidance on the dorsoplantar radiographic projection, confirmed on the lateral, and advanced with the oscillate setting on the drill to reduce risk of broaching the metatarsal cortices. Segmental reduction can be performed with the assistance of percutaneous bone clamps and temporarily-placed Kirschner wires (**Fig. 11**). The

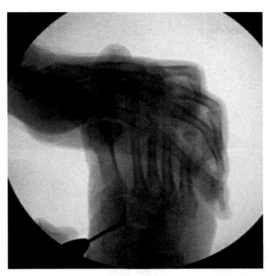

Fig. 7. Fluoroscopy demonstrating naviculocuneiform joint preparation.

guidewires are advanced proximally across the tarsometatarsal arthrodesis site, further proximally across the navicular cuneiform arthrodesis sites, then finally into the talus. When the joints are all prepped, in advance, it can make reduction technically challenging because of the inherent instability imparted by the preparation. Instead, the surgeon can consider preparing the tarsometatarsal joints, introduce the guidewires through the metatarsal heads, across the tarsometatarsal joints into the respective cuneiforms, prepare the naviculocuneiform joints, advance the guidewires more proximally into the navicular, then finally preparing the talonavicular joint,

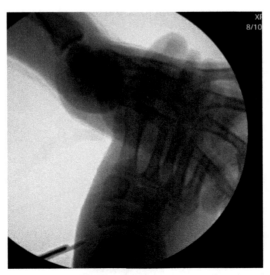

Fig. 8. Fluoroscopy demonstrating percutaneous incisions placed and minimally invasive burr demonstrating talonavicular joint preparation.

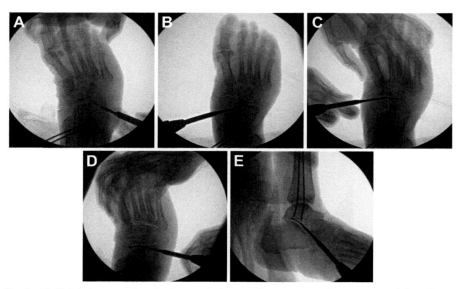

Fig. 9. (*A–E*) Joint preparatory instrumentation used to evacuate the contents of the talona-vicular, naviculocuneiform, and subtalar arthrodesis sites.

and finally advancing the guidewires into the talus. The calcaneocuboid can be trans-fixated in a retrograde approach with the guidewire in the fourth metatarsal. However, if there is any inherent deformity or curvature in the metatarsal, the guidewire may exit the anterior calcaneus prematurely, capturing an insufficient amount of the calcaneus (**Fig. 12**). A separate guidewire, in preparation for screw fixation, can be inserted in retrograde fashion from the anterior cuboid to capture more of the calcaneus. The medial column is ideally stabilized first. Fixation is then introduced from the second and third metatarsal respectively across the midfoot into the talar body, if the

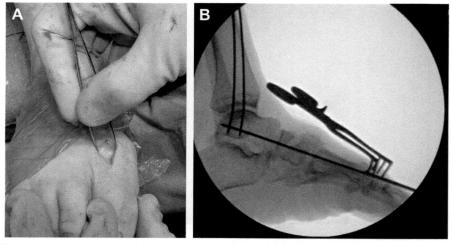

Fig. 10. (*A* and *B*) Dissected first metatarsophalangeal joint in preparation for guidewire.

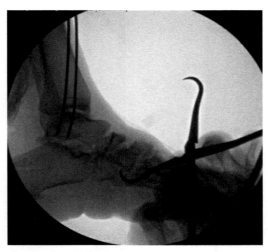

Fig. 11. Utilization of reduction clamps.

trajectory permits. Fixation is then delivered from the fourth metatarsal across the fourth tarsometatarsal arthrodesis site, through the cuboid, and ideally into the calcaneus (**Fig. 13**). The volume of hardware across the talonavicular joint can make dorsal to plantar subtalar joint transfixation logistically challenging and so this is preferentially performed in retrograde fashion from the calcaneus into the talus through a percutaneous incision. All guidewires and transfixation wires are removed and final fluoroscopic images are taken to confirm satisfactory reduction (**Fig. 14**). Skin closure is performed with nonabsorbable suture and the patient is placed in a compression dressing, supplemented with a posterior splint (**Fig. 15**). A circumferential hard cast may not effectively accommodate normal postsurgical edema.

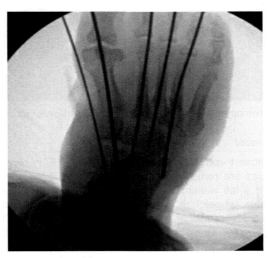

Fig. 12. Fluoroscopy demonstrating guidewires transfixating the first through fourth metatarsals into the talus and calcaneus respectively, prior to delivery of final intramedullary devices.

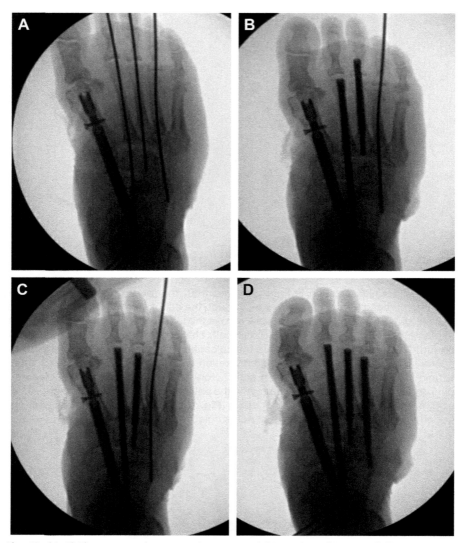

Fig. 13. (*A–D*) Fluoroscopy demonstrating sequential insertion of intramedullary devices.

Postoperative Protocol

Postoperative venous thromboembolic prophylaxis (VTE) is recommended for four to 6 weeks. Sutures are removed in 2 to 4 weeks post surgically and the patient is transitioned into a tall walking boot to remain non-weight bearing for 3 months with a knee scooter, wheelchair, or a rolling walker. During this time, the patient may be passive ankle range of motion exercises once they transition into the boot to reduce VTE risk. Once protected weight bearing formally begins after the third month, and edema has improved, the patient may be fitted for a Charcot Restrained Orthotic Walking (CROW) boot to WBAT in for 6 to 12 months. Some patients, may be transitioned into extra depth molded custom shoes earlier at the physician's discretion.

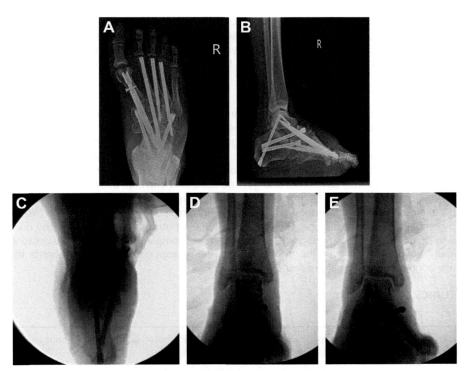

Fig. 14. (*A–E*) Final fluoroscopic and plain film images of reconstruction.

Miscellaneous Considerations

The glycosylated hemoglobin level is an important consideration preoperatively. While Wukich and colleagues have demonstrated that a level greater than 8% has been associated with increased complications, the low morbid approach of the technique has given us the confidence to reconstruct patients with levels approaching 10% as long as prefusion is not compromised.

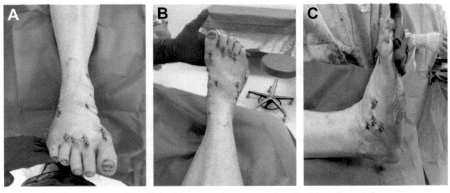

Fig. 15. (*A–C*) Postoperative clinical images demonstrating incisional portals.

With this technique, full reconstruction can be effectively performed within 3 hours, however a Foley catheter is still recommended. This is a procedure that can be performed in the outpatient setting. However, patients with increased comorbidities may still benefit from inpatient admission for observation for a few days.

SUMMARY

Charcot neuroarthropathy is a progressive devastating pathology that alters the quality of life of many patients. There is an inherent level of unpredictability, therefore it is imperative that proper clinical and radiographic work-up is performed to optimized success of limb preservation. Reconstructive surgery should be performed prior to the development of significant complications such as infected or infected ulcerations as this may ultimately save time, energy, and cost, and can improve relative outcomes for patients with midfoot Charcot. Minimally invasive surgical techniques should also be explored as this can reduce soft tissue compromise and optimize osseous healing by respecting natural biology. Patient education is of utmost importance as the duration of treatment and management of unplanned complications can be psychologically overwhelming over the course of treatment, especially in those patients that are considering surgical intervention.

CLINICS CARE POINTS

- Intramedullary fixation spares periosteal perfusion which historically is the dominant source of osseous perfusion.
- Limiting disruption of the soft tissue envelope en route to reconstruction via these minimally invasive approaches is beneficial in this patient population already at risk for poor healing.
- The achilles tendon lengthening in this population is more effective than the gastrocnemius recession.
- The corrective moment for the equinus correction must be performed at the hindfoot and not at the midfoot.

DISCLOSURE

All authors have no financial disclosures to report.

REFERENCES

1. Gupta R. A short history of neuropathic arthropathy. Clin Orthop Relat Res 1993; 296:43–9.
2. Jeffcoate W. The causes of the Charcot syndrome. Clin Podiatr Med Surg 2008; 25(1):29–42, vi.
3. Jordan WR. Neuritic manifestations in diabetes mellitus. Arch Intern Med 1936; 57(2):307–66.
4. Nather A, Bee CS, Huak CY, et al. Epidemiology of diabetic foot problems and predictive factors for limb loss. J Diabetes Complications 2008;22(2):77–82.
5. Kundu AK. Charcot in medical eponyms. J Assoc Physicians India 2004;52: 716–8.
6. McInnes AD. Diabetic foot disease in the United Kingdom: about time to put feet first. J Foot Ankle Res 2012;5:26.

7. Gouveri E, Papanas N. Charcot osteoarthropathy in diabetes: a brief review with an emphasis on clinical practice. World J Diabetes 2011;2:59–65.
8. Singh R, Kishore L, Kaur N. Diabetic peripheral neuropathy: current perspective and future directions. Pharmacol Res 2014;80:21–35.
9. Callaghan B, Feldman E. The metabolic syndrome and neuropathy: therapeutic challenges and opportunities. Ann Neurol 2013;74(3):397–403.
10. Tesfaye S, Stevens LK, Stephenson JM, et al. Prevalence of diabetic peripheral neuropathy and its relation to glycaemic control and potential risk factors: the EURODIAB IDDM Complications Study. Diabetologia 1996;39(11):1377–84.
11. Tesfaye S, Chaturvedi N, Eaton SE, et al. EURODIAB Prospective Complications Study Group. Vascular risk factors and diabetic neuropathy. N Engl J Med 2005; 352(4):341–50.
12. Chantelau E, Onvlee GJ. Charcot foot in diabetes: farewell to the neurotrophic theory. Horm Metab Res 2006;38:361–7.
13. Jeffcoate WJ. Charcot neuro-osteoarthropathy. Diabetes Metab Res Rev 2008; 24(suppl 1):S62–5.
14. Jeffcoate WJ. Abnormalities of vasomotor regulation in the pathogenesis of the acute Charcot foot of diabetes mellitus. Int J Low Extrem Wounds 2005;4(3): 133–7.
15. Kimmerle R, Chantelau E. Weight-bearing intensity produces Charcot deformity in injured neuropathic feet in diabetes. Exp Clin Endocrinol Diabetes 2007;115: 360–4.
16. Vinik AI, Ziegler D. Diabetic cardiovascular autonomic neuropathy. Circulation 2007;115:387–97.
17. Gilbey SG, Walters H, Edmonds ME, et al. Vascular calcification, autonomic neuropathy, and peripheral blood flow in patients with diabetic nephropathy. Diabet Med 1989;6:37–42.
18. Papanas N, Maltezos E. Etiology, pathophysiology and classifications of the diabetic Charcot foot. Diabet Foot Ankle 2013;4:20872.
19. Edmonds ME, Clarke MB, Newton S, et al. Increased uptake of bone radiopharmaceutical in diabetic neuropathy. Q J Med 1985;57:843–55.
20. Sinha S, Munichoodappa C, Kozak GP. Neuro-arthropathy (Charcot joints) in diabetes mellitus. Medicine (Baltim) 1972;51:191–210.
21. Hofbauer LC, Schoppet M. Osteoprotegerin: a link between osteoporosis and arterial calcification? Lancet 2001;358:257–9.
22. Collin-Osdoby P. Regulation of vascular calcification by osteoclast regulatory factors RANKL andosteoprotegerin. Circ Res 2004;95:1046–57.
23. Rosenbaum AJ, DiPreta JA. Classifications in brief: Eichenholtz classification of Charcot arthropathy. author information. Clin Orthop Relat Res 2015;473(3): 1168–71. https://doi.org/10.1007/s11999-014-4059-y.
24. Eichenholtz SN. Charcot joints. Springfield, IL: Charles C. Thomas; 1966.
25. Shibata T, Tada K, Hashizume C. The results of arthrodesis of the ankle for leprotic neuroarthropathy. J Bone Joint Surg Am 1990;72-A:749–56.
26. Ergen FB, Sanverdi SE, Oznur A. Charcot foot in diabetes and an update on imaging. Diabet Foot Ankle 2013;4. https://doi.org/10.3402/dfa.v4i0.21884.eCollection. 2013.
27. Chantelau E, Poll LW. Evaluation of the diabetic Charcot foot by MR imaging or plain radiography—an observational study. Exp Clin Endocrinol Diabetes 2006; 114(8):428–31.
28. Rajbhandari SM, Jenkins RC, Davies C, et al. Charcot neuroarthropathy in diabetes mellitus. Diabetologia 2002;45(8):1085–96.

29. Jones EA, Manaster BJ, May DA, et al. Neuropathic osteoarthropathy: diagnostic dilemmas and differential diagnosis. Radiographics 2000;20(suppl_1):S279–93.
30. Chantelau EA, Richter A. The acute diabetic Charcot foot managed on the basis of magnetic resonance imaging: a review of 71 cases. Swiss Med Wkly 2013;143: w13831.
31. Armstrong DG, Boulton AJM, Bus SA. Diabetic foot ulcers and their recurrence. N Engl J Med 2017;376:2367–75.
32. Broughton G, Janis JE, Attinger CE. The basic science of wound healing. Plast Reconstr Surg 2006;117(7 suppl):12S–34S.
33. Khan NA, Rahim SA, Annad SS, et al. Does the clinical examination predict lower extremity peripheral arterial disease? J Am Med Assoc 2006;295(5):536–46.
34. Marston WA, Davies SW, Armstrong B, et al. Natural history of limbs with arterial insufficiency and chronic ulceration treated without revascularization. J Vasc Surg 2006;44(1):108–14.
35. Attinger CE, Ducic I, Cooper P, et al. The role of intrinsic muscle flaps of the foot for bone coverage in foot and ankle defects in diabetic and nondiabetic patients. Plast Reconstr Surg 2002;110:1047–54.
36. Ramanujam CL, Zgonis T. Versatility of intrinsic muscle flaps for the diabetic Charcot foot. Clin Podiatr Med Surg 2012;29:323–6.
37. Albright RH, Joseph RM, Wukich DK, et al. Is reconstruction of unstable midfoot charcot neuroarthropathy cost effective from a US Payer's perspective? Clin Orthop Relat Res 2020;478(12):2869–88.
38. Doorgakant A, Davies MB. An approach to managing midfoot charcot deformities. Foot Ankle Clin 2020;25(2):319–35.
39. Siddiqui NA, LaPorta GA. Midfoot charcot reconstruction. Clin Podiatr Med Surg 2018;35(4):509–20.
40. Manchanda K, Wallace SB, Ahn J, et al. Charcot midfoot reconstruction: does subtalar arthrodesis or medial column fixation improve outcomes? J Foot Ankle Surg 2020;59(6):1219–23.
41. Lee DJ, Schaffer J, Chen T, et al. Internal versus external fixation of charcot midfoot deformity realignment. Orthopedics 2016;39(4):e595–601.
42. DuBois KS, Cates NK, O'Hara NN, et al. Coronal hindfoot Alignment in midfoot charcot neuroarthropathy. J Foot Ankle Surg 2022;S1067-2516(22):00004–7.
43. LaPorta GA, D'Andelet A. Lengthen, Alignment, and beam technique for midfoot charcot neuroarthropathy. Clin Podiatr Med Surg 2018;35(4):497–507.
44. Lamm BM, Siddiqui NA, Nair AK, et al. Intramedullary foot fixation for midfoot Charcot neuroarthropathy. J Foot Ankle Surg 2012;51(4):531–6.
45. Kwaadu KY. Charcot reconstruction: Understanding and treating the deformed charcot neuropathic arthropathic foot. Clin Podiatr Med Surg 2020;37(2):247–61.
46. Siddiqui NA, LaPorta GA. Minimally invasive bunion correction. Clin Podiatr Med Surg 2018;35(4):387–402.
47. Bocsch P, Markowski H, Rannicher V. Technik und erste ergebnisse der subkutanen distalen metatarsale, I osteotomie. Orthopaedische Praxis 1990;26:51–6.
48. Bocsch P, Wanke S, Legenstein R. Hallux valgus correction by the method of Bocsch: a new technique with a seven-to-ten-year follow-up. Foot Ankle Clin 2000;5(3):485–98.
49. Isham SA. The Reverdin-Isham procedure for the correction of hallux abducto valgus. A distal metatarsal osteotomy procedure. Clin Podiatr Med Surg 1991; 8(1):81–94.
50. Giannini S, Ceccarelli F, Bevoni R, et al. Hallux valgus surgery: the minimally invasive bunion correction (SERI). Tech Foot Ankle Surg 2003;2(1):11–20.

51. Miller RJ. Neuropathic minimally invasive surgeries (NEMESIS): percutaneous diabetic foot surgery and reconstruction. Foot Ankle Clin 2016;21(3):595–627.
52. Crim BE, Lowery NJ, Wukich DK. Internal fixation techniques for midfoot charcot neuroarthropathy in patients with diabetes. Clin Podiatr Med Surg 2011;28(4): 673–85.
53. Perren SM. The biomechanics and biology of internal fixation using plates and nails. Orthopedics 1989;12(1):21–34.

The Navicular Cuneiform Joint

Updates on Avoiding and Managing a Nonunion

Dominick Casciato, DPM, AACFAS[a], Jacob Wynes, DPM, MS, FACFAS[a],*

KEYWORDS

- Flatfoot • Medial column fusion • Midfoot arthritis • Naviculocuneiform fusion

KEY POINTS

- Naviculocuneiform (NC) arthrodesis is a useful procedure for surgical realignment of the midfoot that can be used in isolation or as an adjunct to foot and ankle surgery.
- Nonunion of the NC joint is a known issue that can be managed through understanding of contributing factors and the anatomy of the joint, and through optimization of surgical fixation, leading to successful outcomes.
- Perioperative optimization through appropriate surgical joint preparation and providing metabolic support to the patient may limit the risk of developing a nonunion of the NC joint.

INTRODUCTION

Often performed as an adjunctive procedure with mid- and hindfoot deformity correction, the naviculocuneiform (NC) arthrodesis supplements medial column realignment and stabilization. From conditions such as adult-acquired flatfoot deformity/progressive collapsing foot deformity to primary/post-traumatic arthritis, elimination of motion at this joint enables improvement in foot function. Alongside surgical planning, perioperative consideration of medical history with emphasis on bone metabolism establishes a baseline characterization of bone healing. With nonunion rates ranging from 2.9% to 9.1%, appreciation for such contributing factors leading to nonunion remains imperative.[1–4] Moreover, symptomatic nonunions could necessitate further surgical intervention and ultimately a delay in return to normal ambulation. Thus, understanding the etiology of the nonunion and a focus on its management are paramount to maintaining alignment and pain-free function.

[a] Department of Orthopaedics, Limb Preservation and Deformity Correction Fellowship, University of Maryland School of Medicine, Baltimore, MD, USA
* Corresponding author. University of Maryland Limb Preservation and Deformity Correction Fellowship, 2200 Kernan Drive, Suite 1154c/o Polley Zimnoch, Baltimore, MD 21207.
E-mail address: jwynes@gmail.com

Clin Podiatr Med Surg 40 (2023) 613–621
https://doi.org/10.1016/j.cpm.2023.05.006
0891-8422/23/© 2023 Elsevier Inc. All rights reserved.

ANATOMY

The NC joint serves as a nonessential joint with limited motion, although the facets on its anterior surface provide excursion for the medial and central columns. The medial facet occupies the largest proportion of the NC joint followed by lateral then central facets.[5] Medially, the navicular tuberosity serves as an insertion for the tibialis posterior tendon and plantar calcaneonavicular ligament, often attenuated in planus deformities. Distally, the medial cuneiform provides the insertion site for the tibialis anterior and peroneus longus tendons while the central and lateral cuneiforms assist in providing the keystone for the medial and central rays.[6] The dorsal and plantar surfaces of the navicular are innervated by branches of the dorsalis pedis and medial plantar branch of the posterior tibial artery, respectively, through surface vascular foramina.[7] The cuneiforms are similarly well vascularized, maintaining their vascularity dorsally along the surface via arterial branches of the dorsalis pedis and plantarly from the posterior tibial artery.[8]

INDICATIONS

Preoperative clinical examinations that support NC fusions often reflect periarticular pain secondary to arthritis or medial column collapse. Specifically, the assessment of a rigid, irreducible deformity as seen in medial column collapse, evidenced in progressive collapsing flatfoot deformity, may necessitate a NC fusion as an adjunctive procedure to other osseous procedures. However, an isolated NC fusion, along with a supplementing distal tarsometatarsal fusion, allows for correction and preservation of the essential talonavicular and subtalar joints.[9,10] Weight-bearing radiographic findings may illustrate underlying subchondral cysts and joint space narrowing. Midfoot breach or identification of a center of rotation of angulation (CORA) at the NC joint further indicates fusion. Although advanced imaging beyond weight-bearing radiographs is seldom needed, consideration for other contributing biomechanical or osseous deformity should be given. For example, weight-bearing computed tomography (CT) has shown utility in identifying frontal plane rotation in foot deformities that traditional, non-weight-bearing imaging would fail to identify.[11,12] Notably, attention should be given to patients with a history of diabetes or other neuropathy inciting conditions to rule out Charcot degeneration.

Depending on indication, incision placement may remain isolated or connected to the exposure obtained during other periarticular intervention. Regardless of approach, attention should be made to avoid injury to the tibialis anterior and posterior tendons. Upon visualization of the joint capsule, a capsulotomy is performed, and periarticular soft tissue structures are reflected. A Cobb elevator is introduced into the joint and then distracted. Standard joint preparation is performed, followed with application of an autogenous bone graft harvested from the calcaneus. In revision cases when a greater quantity of bone substrate is desired because of an osseous defect, these authors often request femoral bone marrow harvested with a reamer-irrigator-aspirator. Fixation follows with a combination of screws, staples, or plates. A biomechanical cadaver study found no difference among reduction of the NC joint following lag screw with locking plate for each NC joint, 2 crossed lag screws for each NC joint, and a separate lag screw for each NC joint with bridging locking plates.[13] Plantar plating has been reported for isolated medial naviculocuneiform arthrodesis, with a 15% nonunion rate.[14] The authors' postoperative course consists of non-weight bearing in a posterior splint for 2 weeks then placement into a non-weight-bearing short leg cast for 4 weeks followed by gradual return to range of motion exercises with physical therapy 4 weeks in a CAM (controlled ankle movement) boot. Some flexibility with weight-bearing restriction during the postoperative course is needed to take into account soft tissue and bone healing as assessed clinically and radiographically.

FACTORS TO CONSIDER

Recognizing specific pathology and patient health remain requisite to setting appropriate expectations. For example, NC fusions as part of a medial column super construct in neuropathic arthropathies pose a higher risk of nonunion because of patient comorbidities. Although limited research exists detailing causes of nonunions specific to isolated navicular cuneiform fusions in the elective patient population, surrounding foot and ankle joint fusion data are helpful. Evidenced in mid- and hind-foot arthrodesis, smoking cessation remains important.[15] As a modifiable risk factor, smokers maintain a higher rate of postoperative infection. Laboratory assessment in these individuals includes standard cotinine tests. These authors also recommend preoperative bone metabolism assessment consisting of a 25 dihydroxycholecalciferol laboratory test to assess vitamin D levels.

Although some studies show that nonunion rate among foot and ankle arthrodesis remains equivocal between patients with hypovitaminosis D and those who are sufficient, other research has shown hypovitaminosis D to be associated with a greater risk of nonunion.[16,17] Previous surgeons have employed a 4-week perioperative ergocalciferol supplementation followed by maintenance doses thereafter.[16] Studies have shown cholecalciferol (D3) to be the preferred supplement over ergocalciferol (D2).[18,19] Moreover, as dosing regimens depend on the initial vitamin D levels, therapy should be directed accordingly.[18,20] Although patients with vitamin D deficiency or insufficiency were 8.1 times more likely to experience nonunion compared with those with sufficient levels, other metabolites should be considered.[17] Assisting vitamin D in bone turnover and callous formation, calcium supplementation should be considered.[21] Even further upstream, one may consider parathyroid hormone testing as a litmus test for a patient's bone regeneration ability.[22] Although calcium may be supplemented along with vitamin D; abnormal parathyroid hormone levels may indicate an underlying endocrine disorder and warrant further workup. Other considerations include the current pharmacologic therapy patients are receiving. The short-term use of nonsteroidal anti-inflammatory medication such as ibuprofen and ketorolac in the postoperative period has not been associated with bony non-union.[23]

NONUNION MANAGEMENT

Should pain persist at the site of fusion 8 weeks after surgery, in the absence of an obvious contributing factor such as an open and draining wound or broken hardware, , suspicion for nonunion begins. To supplement this clinical suspicion, basic radiographs along with advanced imaging using CT examination provide sufficient visualization of the presence or absence of osseous bridging across the joint. The type of nonunion should be considered as it assists in determining conservative versus surgical management. For instance, atrophic nonunions do not express osteogenic potential, and should be considered for surgical intervention if symptomatic. Additionally, in these individuals, suspicion for avascular necrosis of the bone proximal and distal to the fusion site should be considered. Although oligotrophic and hypertrophic nonunions present as vascularized nonunions, one should consider extended nonweight bearing as healing potential remains. If the symptomatology includes an erythematous surgical site, septic nonunion may be suspected. If no clinical signs of infection are present, initiation of a bone stimulator may assist. Non-weight bearing accompanied by a pulsed electromagnetic field (PEMF) allows for a noninvasive alternative to implantable devices. Additionally, if not considered preoperatively, vitamin D and calcium assessment with supplementation may prove efficacious. Serial radiographs, and if needed CT scans, then may serve to chronicle healing thereafter. Should healing ultimately stall in a patient with a symptomatic nonunion, revision should follow.

SURGICAL REVISION

Indications for revision of NC arthrodesis include persistent pain at the fusion site that has failed conservative therapy. Asymptomatic nonunions without concern for infection may be monitored so long as subsequent ulceration or deformity does not appear. In the absence of infection, standard debridement of the nonunion site followed by insertion of autogenous graft should be performed. Corticocancellous graft should be considered in situations where medial column shortening is possible secondary to nonunion resection. Adjuncts including demineralized bone matrix, recombinant human bone morphogenetic protein 2, and platelet-rich plasma may assist with healing. With an acceptable safety profile and low complication rate, autologous calcaneal autograft may be harvested and placed into the arthrodesis site.[24] Although technically complicated, arthroscopic revision of the joint has been proven successful.[25] This surgical approach proves effective in minimizing soft tissue dissection and preserving the blood supply to the nonunion site. As with endoscopic approaches, however, complete visualization and removal of soft tissue within the joint following debridement proves difficult.[26]

In the presence of suspected septic nonunion without any obvious surgical site dehiscence, one should assess for warmth to the skin in the immediate area surrounding the operative site. Basic radiographic imaging should then be inspected for loose hardware and any osteitis. Although CT allows for visualization of the arthrodesis site, it provides little sensitivity with regard to any subtle infectious process. Similarly, MRI proves sensitive for osseous changes, especially in the immediate postoperative period; however, it may remain nonspecific for an underlying infection. Radionuclide imaging in the form of white blood cell (WBC) scans (Indium 111 or Ceretec) may provide localization of infection, in this case, around the fusion site. Although reported in traumatic injuries that led to nonunion, leukocyte count (WBC), erythrocyte sedimentation rate, and C-reactive protein were not significant predictors of infection.[27] With continued concern for a symptomatic septic nonunion in the presence of screw/plate loosening and instability, surgical intervention should be considered. Hardware removal followed by arthrodesis site debridement and biopsy, insertion of an antibiotic cement spacer, followed by tailored antibiotic therapy would be appropriate. Once the infection is eradicated and confirmed with bone biopsy, final internal fixation with graft interposition may follow.

NONUNION CASE EXAMPLE

A 52-year-old woman presented to the office with pain to the medial aspect of her right midfoot. She had previously undergone a posterior tibial tendon repair by an outside provider to address painful degenerative changes to her posterior tibial tendon. In the same procedure, she had undergone a medial NC arthrodesis using plate and screw fixation to correct a fault at the NC joint. Her immediate postoperative course was uneventful with the skin incision healing without complication. Over the span of a year, she continued to notice pain to the dorsal-medial aspect of her right midfoot, specifically at the level of the arthrodesis site. Although the incision site remained well-coapted, the right midfoot remained edematous and warm without erythema. She was unable to ambulate without having to sit down after periods of standing to reduce the pain and swelling. Shoe wear modification and pain medication did not provide relief.

The patient had a past medical history of iron deficiency anemia, hypertension, hyperlipidemia, and lumbosacral radiculitis with pain extending to both extremities. She also met the criteria for morbid obesity, with a body mass index (BMI) reported at 46.9. Other than the index naviculocuneiform fusion, she did undergo a laminectomy to her lumbar spine previously. Medications included losartan, ferrous sulfate, hydrochlorothiazide, and a daily multivitamin. She also took oxycodone-acetaminophen, gabapentin, and diclofenac sodium for management for a developed postlaminectomy syndrome. Upon presentation at the office, she showed no systemic signs of infection. Pedal pulses were easily palpable to both feet. She maintained sensation to both lower extremities to the level of the digits. No open wounds or ulcerations were noted to either foot. There was appreciable gross pitting edema noted to the right midfoot without local or radiating erythema. She did exhibit significant tenderness to palpation to the right NC joint at the site of the plate and dorsally. No motion could be elicited at the NC joint, although the proximal and distal joints remained mobile and without pain. Similarly, this pain was reproducible during ambulation, with only rest allowing improvement of her symptoms. She exhibited an antalgic gait on ambulation as she limped to reduce pressure on the right foot.

Radiographic examination revealed an intact plate and screw construct across the medial NC joint. No evidence of hardware loosening or osteolysis was appreciated. There was no osseous bridging seen across this attempted fusion site with evidence of an atrophic nonunion as shown in **Fig. 1**. Diffuse midfoot osteoarthritis still persisted at the remaining naviculocuneiform joints.

At the time of this encounter over 2 years after the index procedure, opportunity for an external bone stimulator had passed. Considering the patient had exhausted conservative management of the nonunion including periods of physical therapy, pain medication, and custom orthotics, the patient shared interest in a revision procedure. Because of the combined nonunion and arthritis to the remaining NC joint, the patient was agreeable to and consented for a hardware removal and attempted revision arthrodesis of the entire joint. Furthermore, to assist with healing, calcaneal autograft was planned. Preoperatively, the patient was ordered vitamin D and parathyroid

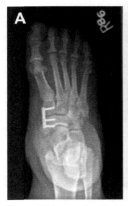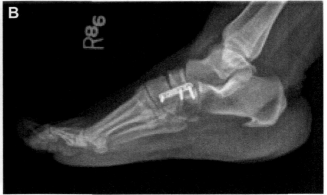

Fig. 1. (A) Anterior-posterior and (B) lateral radiographs of nonunion upon presentation.

hormone (PTH) tests; however, she did not complete at the time of the procedure. Despite this, she was given a vitamin D supplement in the immediate perioperative period through the postoperative phase.

The patient underwent surgical intervention first with calcaneal autograft harvesting. The NC joint was visualized through a midmedial approach to allow for hardware removal. After the previous plate and screws were removed, the nonunion site was resected, and deep bone specimens were sent for culture and histopathological examination. The site was then further prepared using a standard technique with osteotomes, burr, and subchondral fenestration. The arthrodesis site was then packed with calcaneal autograft and bone morphogenic protein (BMP2). With the foot held in neutral and simulated weight bearing, the joint temporarily was held in a reduced position with k-wires and fixed with 3 × 4.0 mm headless screws. Order of screw placement consisted of fixation of the intermediate then lateral cuneiform followed by the medial cuneiform into the navicular. The incision site was closed with suture and the foot placed in a Robert Jones splint.

She followed up 1 week after the procedure without any evidence of wound healing or hardware complications. The resulting negative bone cultures were shared with the patient. Moreover, the histopathology assessment, detailing articular cartilage and synovium with mild degenerative changes was discussed. Casting of the operative extremity occurred 2 weeks postoperatively. She continued with routine bone healing through the first month following the procedure as shown in **Fig. 2**. Subsequent placement into a CAM boot 6 weeks postoperatively while maintaining non-weight bearing and initiation of physical therapy ensued. Full weight bearing was allowed at 12 weeks. At the last follow-up appointment 5 months after the procedure, consolidation of the NC joint was appreciated radiographically without residual pain at the arthrodesis site (**Fig. 3**).

DISCUSSION

In conclusion, NC arthrodesis provides a powerful means of deformity correction whether isolated or in conjunction with fore- and hindfoot reconstruction. Despite best attempts, nonunions pose an ever-present outcome and should be managed in an algorithmic manner to efficiently address the operative site. As seen in elective

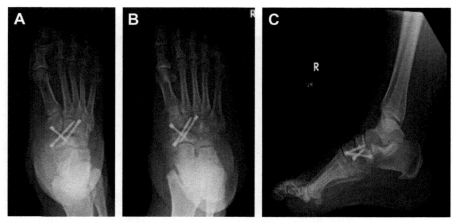

Fig. 2. (*A*) Anterior-posterior, (*B*) medial oblisque, and (*C*) lateral radiographic projections showing healing 1 month following revision NC fusion.

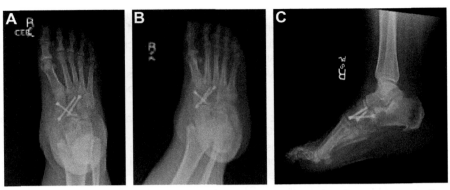

Fig. 3. (*A*) Anterior-posterior, (*B*) medial oblique, and (*C*) lateral radiographic projections showing healing 5 months following revision NC fusion.

foot and ankle surgery, assessing modifiable and metabolic risk factors before surgical intervention proves useful in minimizing nonunions. If a symptomatic nonunion should present, determining underlying etiology allows one to determine conservative versus surgical management. If healing continues as seen with radiography, bone stimulation and nutritional supplementation may avoid revision. When intervention is indicated, continuation of sound arthrodesis principles in providing stable fixation between bony segments with supplementary grafts optimizes the revision.

CLINICS CARE POINTS

- Appropriate fixation and attention to meticulous intraoperative alignment is important in avoiding NC arthrodesis nonunion.
- Repair of symptomatic nonunion of the NC joint should involve the use of autogenous bone grafting and revision of hardware with stable surgical fixation.
- Vitamin D optimization and smoking cessation have demonstrated efficacy in the prevention and management of NC nonunion.
- It is imperative to evaluate the etiology of the nonunion, as this can influence surgical decision making such as discerning atrophic versus hypertrophic nonunion and ruling out infection.

DISCLOSURE

Neither author reports conflicts of interest or financial disclosures as they pertain to the drafting or content of this article.

REFERENCES

1. Chu AK, Wilson MD, Lee J, et al. The incidence of nonunion of the naviculocuneiform joint arthrodesis: a systematic review. J Foot Ankle Surg 2019;58:545–9.
2. Steiner CS, Gilgen A, Zwicky L, et al. Combined subtalar and naviculocuneiform fusion for treating adult acquired flatfoot deformity with medial arch collapse at the level of the naviculocuneiform joint. Foot Ankle Int 2019;40:42–7.
3. Gerrity M, Williams M. Naviculocuneiform arthrodesis in adult flatfoot: a case series. J Foot Ankle Surg 2019;58:352–6.

4. Ajis A, Geary N. Surgical technique, fusion rates, and planovalgus foot deformity correction with naviculocuneiform fusion. Foot Ankle Int 2014;35:232–7.

5. Renner K, McAlister JE, Galli MM, et al. Anatomic description of the naviculocuneiform articulation. J Foot Ankle Surg 2017;56:19–21.

6. Casciato D, Yancovitz S, Olivová J, et al. Anatomic description of the distal and intercuneiform articulations: a cadaveric study. J Foot Ankle Surg 2021;60:1137–43.

7. Golano P, Fariñas O, Sáenz I. The anatomy of the navicular and periarticular structures. Foot Ankle Clin 2004;9:1–23.

8. Kraus JC, McKeon KE, Johnson JE, et al. Intraosseous and extraosseous blood supply to the medial cuneiform: implications for dorsal opening wedge plantar-flexion osteotomy. Foot Ankle Int 2014;35:394–400.

9. Greisberg J, Assal M, Hansen ST Jr, et al. Isolated medial column stabilization improves alignment in adult-acquired flatfoot. Clin Orthop Relat Res 2005;435:197–202.

10. Greisberg J, Hansen ST Jr, Sangeorzan B. Deformity and degeneration in the hindfoot and midfoot joints of the adult acquired flatfoot. Foot Ankle Int 2003;24:530–4.

11. Lalevée M, Barbachan Mansur NS, Dibbern K, et al. Coronal plane rotation of the medial column in hallux valgus: a retrospective case-control study. Foot Ankle Int 2022;43(8):1041–8.

12. Bernasconi A, De Cesar Netto C, Siegler S, et al. Weightbearing CT assessment of foot and ankle joints in pes planovalgus using distance mapping. Foot Ankle Surg 2022;28(6):775–84.

13. Kuestermann H, Ettinger S, Yao D, et al. Biomechanical evaluation of naviculocuneiform fixation with lag screw and locking plates. Foot Ankle Surg 2021;27:911–9.

14. Wininger AE, Klavas DM, Gardner SS, et al. Plantar plating for medial naviculocuneiform arthrodesis in progressive collapsing foot deformity. Foot Ankle Orthop 2022;7. 24730114221088517.

15. Allport J, Ramaskandhan J, Siddique MS. Nonunion rates in hind- and midfoot arthrodesis in current, ex-, and nonsmokers. Foot Ankle Int 2021;42:582–8.

16. Ebben BJ, Brooks AE, Gaio NM, et al. Vitamin D management and nonunion in elective foot and ankle arthrodesis. Foot & Ankle Orthopaedics 2020;5. https://doi.org/10.1177/2473011420S00197.

17. Moore KR, Howell MA, Saltrick KR, et al. Risk factors associated with nonunion after elective foot and ankle reconstruction: a case-control study. J Foot Ankle Surg 2017;56:457–62.

18. Holick MF, Binkley NC, Bischoff-Ferrari HA, et al. Evaluation, treatment, and prevention of vitamin D deficiency: an Endocrine Society clinical practice guideline. J Clin Endocrinol Metab 2011;96:1911–30.

19. Armas LAG, Hollis BW, Heaney RP. Vitamin D2 is much less effective than vitamin D3 in humans. J Clin Endocrinol Metab 2004;89:5387–91.

20. Patton CM, Powell AP, Patel AA. Vitamin D in orthopaedics. J Am Acad Orthop Surg 2012;20:123–9.

21. Fischer V, Haffner-Luntzer M, Amling M, et al. Calcium and vitamin D in bone fracture healing and post-traumatic bone turnover. Eur Cell Mater 2018;35:365–85.

22. Wojda SJ, Donahue SW. Parathyroid hormone for bone regeneration. J Orthop Res 2018;36:2586–94.

23. Hassan MK, Karlock LG. The effect of post-operative NSAID administration on bone healing after elective foot and ankle surgery. Foot Ankle Surg 2020;26: 457–63.
24. Law RW, Langan TM, Consul DW, et al. Safety profile associated with calcaneal autograft harvesting using a reaming graft harvester. Foot Ankle Int 2020;41: 1487–92.
25. Lui TH. Arthroscopic revision arthrodesis for non-union of the naviculocuneiform joint: a case report. J Orthop Surg 2015;23:267–9.
26. Kim SJ, Shin SJ, Yang KH, et al. Endoscopic bone graft for delayed union and nonunion. Yonsei Med J 2000;41:107–11.
27. Brinker MR, Macek J, Laughlin M, et al. Utility of common biomarkers for diagnosing infection in nonunion. J Orthop Trauma 2021;35:121–7.

Medial Double Arthrodesis Through Single Approach

Edgar Sy, DPM, AACFAS[a],*, Matthew D. Sorensen, DPM, FACFAS[b,1]

KEYWORDS

- Arthrodesis • Medial • Double • Flatfoot • PTTD • Arthritis • Subtalar
- Talonavicular

KEY POINTS

- The medial double arthrodesis has gained popularity as an effective procedure that avoids potential sequelae such as calcaneocuboid joint (CCJ) nonunion or lateral wound dehiscence that has been reported following a triple arthrodesis.
- Execution of a medial double in contrast to a triple arthrodesis includes benefits to the patient such as decreased soft tissue complications with a single incision, decreased osseous nonunion complications of attempted CCJ fusion, decreased operative time, preservation of the lateral column length, and decreased cost.
- The medial double arthrodesis spares the CCJ joint that allows motion in an effort to dissipate the stresses on the ankle and midfoot joints to a considerable extent, thus aiding in prevention of adjacent joint arthritis and allows for accommodation of uneven surfaces.
- Avascular necrosis is a postoperative complication, although viewed as a rare event, that remains possible in double or triple hindfoot arthrodesis—only the lateral portion of the body of the talus is nourished by the tarsal sinus artery, which is preserved in the medial approach.

INTRODUCTION

Triple arthrodesis is a time-tested procedure toward primary salvage in the context of posterior tibial tendon dysfunction (PTTD), symptomatic rigid and severe hindfoot malalignment, end-stage degenerative and posttraumatic arthritis, and sequelae of paralytic diseases. Triple arthrodesis consists of arthrodesis of the subtalar joint (STJ) and both transverse tarsal joints, talonavicular and calcaneocuboid joints (TNJ and CCJ). This technique was initially described in 1923 by Ryerson for severe congenital or paralytic deformities where transosseous catgut suture and cast

[a] Weil Foot & Ankle Institute, Chicago, IL, USA; [b] OrthoIllnois, Chicago, IL, USA
[1] Present address: 650 South Randall Road, Algonquin, IL 60102.
* Corresponding author. 10041 Pines Boulevard suite e, Pembroke Pines, FL 33024.
E-mail address: EdgarFSy@gmail.com

Clin Podiatr Med Surg 40 (2023) 623–632
https://doi.org/10.1016/j.cpm.2023.05.005
0891-8422/23/Published by Elsevier Inc.
podiatric.theclinics.com

immobilization was historically used with the procedure.[1] The traditional incisional approach to the procedure is to use a dual incisional approach: one incision on the medial aspect of the foot to access the TNJ and a second incision to the lateral aspect in effort to access both the subtalar and calcaneocuboid joint (CCJ). Today, the indication for hindfoot arthrodesis is applied to correct painful deformities and arthritic joints, such as advanced cases of adult-acquired flatfoot secondary to ligament collapse and insufficiency of the posterior tibial tendon. Although the triple arthrodesis is an effective and reliable outcome procedure, the popularity of a medial double arthrodesis (fusion of subtalar joint [STJ] and TNJ) has increased, as more research has indicated reliable results with high osseous union rate and additional benefits of sparing the CCJ.

Execution of a medial double in contrast to a triple arthrodesis includes benefits to the patient such as decreased soft tissue complications with a single incision, decreased osseous nonunion complications of attempted CCJ fusion, decreased operative time, preservation of the lateral column length, and decreased cost. These are each important factors in consideration of the medial double (**Fig. 1**). Through a single medial incision, studies have consistently shown surgeons maintain the ability to adequately and accurately reduce deformity both radiographically, functionally, and clinically.[1] O'Malley and colleagues using a cadaver model demonstrated that restoration of arch height and forefoot rotation did not require the addition of the CCJ to the corrective arthrodesis.[2] Furthermore, Berlet and colleagues demonstrated CCJ osteoarthritis may be improved at least one grade after double arthrodesis due to functional arthrodiastasis subsequent to deformity correction of TNJ and STJ.[3] Investigators have found indications for calcaneocuboid arthrodesis limited to stage 4 "bone on bone" arthritis, painful unstable joint mechanics, and/or frank subluxation at the CCJ.[4] Regardless of the surgeon's chosen procedural selection, precise hindfoot realignment is crucial to the outcome of the procedure.

Multiple hindfoot joint arthrodesis is the traditional treatment of stage 3 and 4 adult-acquired flatfoot deformity. The nidus for pes-plano-valgus deformity in adults is thought to originate from a compromised tibialis posterior tendon, resulting in posterior tibial tendon dysfunction and insufficiency. This tendon serves as an important dynamic stabilizer of the medial arch of the foot; the arch begins to collapse and flatten as the tendon fails. This progressive deformity places stress on adjacent structures in the foot and ankle, such as the spring ligament, and deltoid ligament complex, which has been shown to progress into attenuation or rupture. Patients with PTTD may slowly progress to a severe and rigid deformity secondary to joint collapse associated

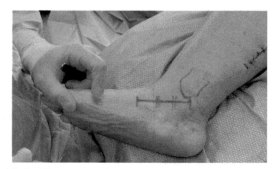

Fig. 1. Medial double incision approach.

with soft-tissue failure and subsequent degenerative change to joints that are functioning abnormally. This progression is characterized by dorsolateral subluxation of the navicular on the talus, lateral column shortening in relation to the medical column, fixed supination of the forefoot, and potential arthritis of the hindfoot joints.[5] PTTD was originally classified by Johnson and Strom into 3 stages, according to the progression of deformity, later modified by Myerson to include a fourth stage. Stage III is defined by a rigid deformity that is not passively correctable; the focus of operative intervention should shift from soft tissue techniques and corrective osteotomies to hindfoot arthrodesis procedures.

ADVANTAGES

The medial double arthrodesis has gained popularity as an effective procedure that avoids potential sequelae such as CCJ nonunion or lateral wound dehiscence that has been reported following a triple arthrodesis.[5] Sparing the CCJ avoids both soft tissue and osseous complications, as the inherent risk of osseous nonunion reported as high as 17.2% and soft tissue infection reported at a 10% rate.[6,7] In addition, avoiding fusion of the CCJ preserves the lateral column length. By foregoing the removal of the articular cartilage of the lateral column, the lateral column length is preserved, which in turn facilitates reduction and correction of the abducted forefoot in the planovalgus deformity.[5,8,9] Also, a cadaver study on the normal foot by Jeng and colleagues showed that 91% of the STJ and 91% of the TNJ could be prepared by the medial approach.[10]

The union rates for this medial single incision have been predictable and comparable with the dual incision approach. Anand and colleagues demonstrated a successful STJ and TNJ union rate of 89% with a mean follow-up of 24 months.[5] In 3 different studies, Knupp and colleagues, Philippot and colleagues, Fadle and colleagues, and Brilhault reported a 32/32 (100%), 14/14 (100%), 23/23 (100%), and 15/15 (100%) union rate after double arthrodesis, respectively.[4,8,11,12] Tejero and colleagues published the largest cohort (67 feet) of medial double arthrodesis with the most extended mean follow-up to date (6.6 years). They reported a result of complete union in 60 out of 67 feet (89%). Four out of the seven of these nonunions developed as asymptomatic TNJ pseudoarthrosis and required no additional surgery.[13] However, these results contradict the findings of another retrospective, comparative study by Burrus and colleagues who reported unfavorable outcomes in the double arthrodesis group. Four of the nine (44%) medial double arthrodesis had TN nonunion, 6 (67%) had hardware failure, and reported 5 (56%) lost hindfoot deformity correction.[14] Recently, Cates and colleagues published systematic review with a total of 13 articles (343 subjects) to investigate fusion rates and mean time to fusion in double and triple arthrodesis. They found an overall fusion rate of 91.75% (289/315) for double arthrodesis compared with 92.86% (26/28) triple arthrodesis fusion rate with a mean time of 17.96 and 16.70 weeks.

It has proved that among the 3 joints, the position of the TNJ is considered the keystone and critical for midfoot and hindfoot alignment.[5,9] A classic article demonstrated in a cadaveric study performing isolated and combined hindfoot arthrodesis that fusion of the TNJ essentially eliminated motion at the other 2 joints, indicating that fusing this joint should maintain any hindfoot realignment. At baseline, the CCJ has an average 14.7° of motion, the least of all the hindfoot joints; however, Astion and colleagues demonstrated once the TNJ was fused motion through the CCJ will be only approximately 2°.[15] A properly positioned isolated arthrodesis of the TNJ has been shown to be effective in correcting all of the deformities of a flexible planovalgus foot, as shown by O'Malley[2] and Harper and Tisdel.[16] However, adequate correction for frontal plane rigid planovalgus foot deformity cannot be achieved with just isolated TNJ arthrodesis; therefore, STJ arthrodesis is required for coronal deformity for a well-positioned plantigrade foot.[4,5] Studies have shown that over time the joints adjacent to the triple arthrodesis, such as the ankle and midfoot joints, will demonstrate increased secondary arthritic degeneration or "transfer arthritis." Adjacent joint midfoot and ankle joint degenerative changes because of abnormal stresses after triple arthrodesis range from 30% to 50%. The medial double arthrodesis spares the CCJ joint that allows motion in an effort to dissipate the stresses on the ankle and midfoot joints to a considerable extent, thus aiding in prevention of adjacent joint arthritis.[5] The few degrees of residual mobility that remains in the lateral column of the foot through the open CCJ may protect these adjacent joints by dissipating the forces during ambulation. This protective effect on adjacent joints is also supported by Sammarco and colleagues and Hyer and colleagues[17,18] Tejero and colleagues reported that only 4 out of 67 (5.9%) feet with double arthrodesis developed deformity progression and required ankle arthrodesis at 6.6 years of follow-up.[13]

There has been effort toward the preservation of the CCJ and 4 of 5 tarsometatarsal joints to allow for accommodation of uneven surfaces.[3] Through the medial double, the CCJ is preserved as a mobile adaptor but also in effort to decrease the long-term morbidity of the adjacent joints, in contrast to long-term data available for the ankle after triple arthrodesis.[3] The CCJ has often been noted to distract and decompress with the abduction correction achieved through medial double fusion. The arthrodiastasis effect at the CCJ has been shown to allow remodeling of sclerosis and arthrosis radiographically. Berlet and colleagues investigated 20 feet with a mean follow-up of 9.2 months to report distention of the CCJ, which increased joint space and improvement of at least 1 grade of arthritis in 50% of patients with mild to moderate arthritis. They reported an average of 9 months to radiographically measure subchondral bone changes.[3] Although historically there were concerns of CCJ arthritis as a long-term complication of medial hindfoot arthritis, Fadle and colleagues showed that none of the patients in the medial-double arthrodesis group developed any arthritic changes to the CCJ or lateral pain at 1 year postoperatively.[4]

Correction of hindfoot cause has the potential to uncover or create a secondary ankle valgus deformity due to extended medial dissection and possible disruption of the deltoid ligament. Two potential rationales for the occurrence of postoperative ankle valgus have been postulated. First, in the case of a medial double approach, portions of the deltoid ligament complex are resected to gain access to the STJ middle and posterior facets. Although this ligament is repaired during closure, it is possible that weakening the deltoid ligament complex can occur and subsequent ankle valgus may result. Secondly, in the case of triple arthrodesis, the fused hindfoot with a slight or more significant level of residual valgus may give rise to a stronger lever arm against the medial soft tissue structures causing them to fail as valgus moment forces are dissipated to the ankle. Hyer and colleagues compared triple and medial double arthrodesis for progression of ankle valgus postoperatively with a mean follow-up of 8.75 months, in which they found the odds of having an increase in ankle valgus for patients in the triple group was 3.64 times that for patients in the double group, as the medial double arthrodesis was protective against the development of ankle valgus postoperatively.[18]

Avascular necrosis is a postoperative complication, although viewed as a rare event, that remains possible in double or triple hindfoot arthrodesis. Studies show that peritalar vascularization including the tarsal and deltoid arteries is responsible for 3-quarters of the nutrition to the talar body. Only the lateral portion of the body of the talus is nourished by the tarsal sinus artery, which is preserved in the medial approach.[19] Miller and colleagues demonstrated the existence of a rich intra- and extraosseous anastomotic network, which could explain the viability of the talus even when only one of the arteries is preserved.[20] When engaging the single-incision medial double arthrodesis, Rohm and colleagues developed avascular necrosis in only 3 of 96 feet.[21] Phisitkul and colleagues compared the degree of vascular injuries between the single-medial-incision approach and the 2-incision approach for hindfoot arthrodesis. The single-medial-incision approach damaged the deltoid artery in 86% and tarsal canal artery in 100% of the specimens. The double incisional approach preserved the deltoid artery.[22] It is important for surgeons during dissection that access to the deep portion of the deltoid ligament should be avoided, preserving as much as possible the integrity of the medial ligament complex to minimize risks.

An additional benefit of performing a medial double arthrodesis and sparing the calcaneocuboid joint is reduction in operative time. Fadle and colleagues demonstrated a significantly shorter mean operative time by nearly 35 minutes in the arthrodesis group, from 55.77 minutes versus 91.6 minutes.[4] Galli and colleagues reported similar findings as the mean procedure time was significantly shorter in double arthrodesis than triple arthrodesis, 84 versus 104 minutes. Moreover, the implants for triple arthrodesis cost, on average, 2.4 times those for double arthrodesis.[23]

Double arthrodesis has a low risk of soft tissue complications and presents with satisfactory functional results. Ferreira and colleagues had a patient satisfaction rate of 79% with 18 patients, which is considered the result of treatment excellent or good, which is similar to Anand and colleagues that reported an overall satisfactory rate of 78%.[1,5] A similar finding was reported by Rohm and colleagues where they reported a 66% satisfactory rate, which is considered good or very good outcome.[21] Anand and colleagues after evaluating 18 patients found 39% were very satisfied, 39% were satisfied with minor reservations, and 22% were dissatisfied at the end of follow-up. These investigators considered that these results were not encouraging enough to recommend the adoption of double arthrodesis as an alternative to triple arthrodesis.[5] However, other studies evaluating triple arthrodesis have reported results similar to those obtained in double arthrodesis. Sangeorzan and colleagues and Stegeman and colleagues, respectively, obtained results considered good by 77% and 74% of patients, respectively.[24–27] Walker and colleagues included 13 studies in a systematic review toward evaluating the outcome of 481 patients with deformities of various causes who underwent triple arthrodesis using a 2-incision approach. Outcome was good in 74% of patients, fair in 18%, and poor in 8%.[6]

TECHNIQUES

Procedures are typically performed with the patient in the supine position, using a pneumatic thigh tourniquet. Bone marrow aspirate is routinely procured as a benign ancillary procedure toward increasing stem cell count in the fusion mass and increasing fusion rates. Other ancillary soft-tissue procedures such as posterior muscle group lengthening can be performed as needed in the same sitting.

For the medial double approach an incision is made from the inframedial malleolus, following the course of the posterior tibial tendon superiorly all the way to distal to the navicular tuberosity (see **Fig. 1**). Dissection is carefully carried deep, taking care to cauterize and retract tributaries to the medial marginal vein and retract the saphenous nerve. The posterior tibial tendon sheath is then identified and incision is made through

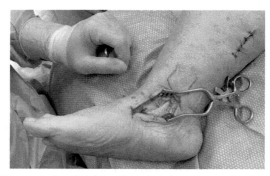

Fig. 2. Access to the posterior tibial tendon sheath and superior border of the tendon noted.

the sheath to gain access to the TNJ and STJ capsules (**Fig. 2**). The PTT tendon repair or resection can also be addressed through this incision. Once access has been gained to the TNJ, a vertical incision in line with the TNJ is made through the capsule (**Fig. 3**). That capsular incision is followed inferiorly and posteriorly along the inferior border of the talar head and neck directly into the middle facet of the STJ. Once the middle facet has been identified, the capsular incision is carried further proximal into the posterior facet region of the STJ (**Fig. 4**). Care is taken to reflect only a minimal amount of deltoid ligament fibers to mitigate postoperative, iatrogenic attenuation. The cervical ligament is then identified through the medial approach and is resected to allow for adequate distraction of the STJ and access for debridement of both the posterior and middle facets. The investigators prefer the use of a static distraction device to maintain predictable access to the joint surfaces for debridement. A combination of curettage and osteotome debridement is used to remove all residual cartilage from both facets down to subchondral bleeding bone. The corresponding surfaces of

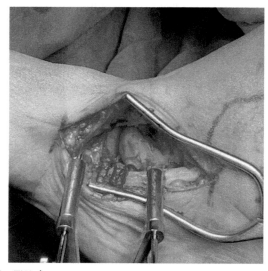

Fig. 3. Access to the TNJ shown.

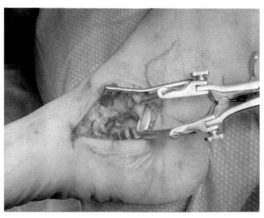

Fig. 4. Visualization of the middle and posterior facets of the STJ noted.

each facet are then fenestrated using a 2.0 mm drill bit as well as small osteotome in an effort to provide a bleeding bone surface for fusion (**Fig. 5**).

Next, attention is directed to the medial aspect of the TNJ where the previously arthrotomy was performed to gain access to the joint. Again, a static distraction device is used to maintain distraction for joint debridement. The exact same debridement process is engaged for the TNJ as for the STJ.

Once confidence is attained that all joint surfaces have been adequately debrided, autograft or synthetic graft may be placed within each joint to aid in ultimate fusion. Next, the TNJ is reduced, as the most powerful joint for reduction of hindfoot deformity in all 3 planes, and provisionally pinned in its reduced position. The investigators prefer the use of cannulated lag screws or dynamic compression staples or locked plating or a combination thereof for fixation across the TNJ. Once the TNJ is stabilized, the STJ will be reduced in all 3 planes and needs to be fixated using 6.5 mm or 5.5 mm lag

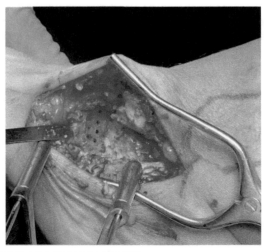

Fig. 5. Access and joint prep shown to the TNJ.

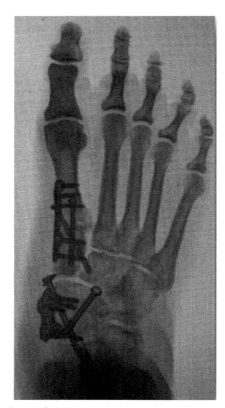

Fig. 6. Postoperative radiographs.

screws to maintain position and provide a level of compression across the fusion, providing an invitation for the fusion mass to heal (**Figs. 6** and **7**).

Intraoperative fluoroscopy should be used throughout the procedures to ensure adequate reduction of deformity as well as accurate placement of chosen implants.

Once the TNJ and STJ have been definitively fixated, other soft tissue procedures can commence based on surgeon preference.

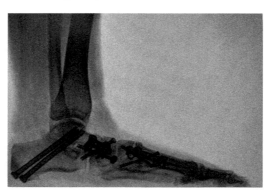

Fig. 7. Lateral view postoperative films.

CLINICS CARE POINTS

- It has been proved that among the 3 joints, the position of the TNJ is considered the keystone and critical for midfoot and hindfoot alignment.

- Through the medial double, the calcaneocuboid joint is preserved as a mobile adaptor but also in effort to decrease the long-term morbidity of the adjacent joints, in contrast to long-term data available for the ankle after triple arthrodesis.

- Portions of the deltoid ligament complex are resected to gain access to the STJ middle and posterior facets. Although this ligament is repaired during closure, it is possible that weakening the deltoid ligament complex can occur and subsequent ankle valgus may result.

DISCLOSURE

The authors have nothing to disclose.

REFERENCES

1. Ferreira GF, Nava N, Durigon TS, et al. Double hindfoot arthrodesis using a single-incision medial approach in the correction of adult-acquired flatfoot deformity: a case series, International Orthopedics, 45 (9), 2021, 2375–2381.
2. O'Malley MJ, Deland JT, Lee K-T. Selective hindfoot arthrodesis for the treatment of adult acquired flatfoot deformity: an in vitro study. Foot Ankle Int 1995;16: 411–7.
3. Berlet GC, Hyer CF, Scott RT, et al. Medial double arthrodesis with lateral column sparing and arthrodiastasis: a radiographic and medical record review, J Foot Ankle Surg, 54 (3), 2015, 441–444.
4. Fadle AA, El-Adly W, Attia AK, et al. Double versus triple arthrodesis for adult-acquired flatfoot deformity due to stage III posterior tibial tendon insufficiency: a prospective comparative study of two cohorts, International Orthopedics, 45 (9), 2021, 2219–2229.
5. Anand P, Nunley JA, DeOrio JK. Single-incision medial approach for double arthrodesis of hindfoot in posterior tibialis tendon dysfunction. Foot Ankle Int 2013;34(3):338–44.
6. Walker R, Francis R, Singh S, et al. Death of the triple arthrodesis? Orthop Traumatol 2015;29(5):324–33.
7. Klassen LJ, Shi E, Weinraub GM, et al. Comparative nonunion rates in triple arthrodesis. J Foot Ankle Surg 2018;57(6):1154–6.
8. Knupp M, Schuh R, Stufkens SAS, et al. Subtalar and talonavicular arthrodesis through a single medial approach for the correction of severe planovalgus deformity. J Bone Jt Surg Br 2009;91(5):612–5.
9. DeVries JG, Scharer B. Hindfoot deformity corrected with double versus triple arthrodesis: radiographic comparison. J Foot Ankle Surg 2015;54(3):424–7.
10. Jeng CL, Tankson CJ, Myerson MS. The single medial approach to triple arthrodesis: a cadaver study. Foot Ankle Int 2006;27:1122–5.
11. Philippot R, Wegrzyn J, Besse JL. Arthrodesis of the subtalar and talonavicular joints through a medial surgical approach: a series of 15 cases. Arch Orthop Trauma Surg 2010;130:599–603.
12. Brilhault J. Single medial approach to modified double arthrodesis in rigid flatfoot with lateral deficient skin. Foot Ankle Int 2009;30(1):21–6.

13. Tejero S, Carranza-Pérez-Tinao A, Zambrano-Jiménez MD, et al. Minimally invasive technique for stage III adult-acquired flatfoot deformity: a mid- to long-term retrospective study. Int Orthop 2021;45:217–23.
14. Burrus MT, Werner BC, Carr JB, et al. Increased failure rate of modified double arthrodesis compared with triple arthrodesis for rigid pes planovalgus. J Foot Ankle Surg 2016;55:1169–74.
15. Astion DJ, Deland JT, Otis JC, et al. Motion of the hindfoot after simulated arthrodesis. J Bone Joint Surg Am 1997;79:241–6.
16. Harper MC, Tisdel CL. Talonavicular arthrodesis for the painful adult acquired flatfoot. Foot Ankle Int 1996;17:658–61.
17. Sammarco VJ, Magur EG, Sammarco GJ, et al. Arthrodesis of the subtalar and talonavicular joints for correction of symptomatic hindfoot malalignment. Foot Ankle Int 2006;27:661–6.
18. Hyer CF, Galli MM, Scott RT, et al. Ankle valgus after hindfoot arthrodesis: a radiographic and chart comparison of the medial double and triple arthrodeses, J Foot Ankle Surg, 53 (1), 2014, 55–58.
19. Mulfnger GL, Trueta J. The blood supply of the talus. J Bone Joint Surg Br 1970; 52(1):160–7.
20. Miller et al. demonstrated the existence of a rich intra- and extra-osseous anastomotic network, which could explain the viability of the talus even with only one of the arteries preserved.
21. Rohm J, Zwicky L, Horn Lang T, et al. Mid- to long-term outcome of 96 corrective hindfoot fusions in 84 patients with rigid fatfoot deformity. Bone Joint Lett J 2015; 97-B(5):668–74.
22. Phisitkul P, Haugsdal J, Vaseenon T, et al. Vascular disruption of the talus: comparison of two approaches for triple arthrodesis. Foot Ankle Int 2013;34(4): 568–74.
23. Galli MM, Scott RT, Bussewitz BW, et al. A retrospective comparison of cost and efficiency of the medial double and dual incision triple arthrodeses. Foot Ankle Spec 2014;7:32–6.
24. Sangeorzan BJ, Smith D, Veith R, et al. Triple arthrodesis using internal fixation in treatment of adult foot disorders. Clin Orthop Relat Res 1993;294:299–307.
25. Stegeman M, Anderson PG, Louwerens JWK. Triple arthrodesis of the hindfoot, a short term prospective outcome study. Foot Ankle Surg 2006;12(2):71–7.
26. So E, Reb CW, Larson DR, et al. Medial double arthrodesis: technique guide and tips, J Foot Ankle Surg, 57 (2), 2018, 364–369.
27. Jones CK, Nunley JA. Osteonecrosis of the lateral aspect of the talar dome after triple arthrodesis. A report of three cases. J Bone Joint Surg Am 1999;81(8): 1165–9.

Revision of Subtalar Joint Arthrodesis

Considerations for Bone Grafting, Fixation Constructs, and Three-Dimensional Printing

Ryan J. Lerch, DPM[a], Amar Gulati, DPM[b],
Peter D. Highlander, DPM, MS[a],*

KEYWORDS

- Subtalar arthrodesis • Fusion • Nonunion • Revision • 3D printing • Bone grafting

KEY POINTS

- Although relatively high satisfaction and union rates have been reported for isolated subtalar joint arthrodesis, questions still remain as to graft options, fixation techniques, and revisions.
- It is the authors' recommendation that in the setting of failed subtalar joint arthrodesis, to use autograft with intramedullary nailing as a revision construct.
- Isolated subtalar joint arhtrodesis has proven to be a predictable and successful option for treatment of various foot and ankle pathologies.

INTRODUCTION/HISTORY/DEFINITIONS/BACKGROUND

It is well known that foot and ankle surgery in the United States has been increasing for the past couple of decades as shown in the literature. In a period of 17 years, Best and colleagues[1] demonstrated using National Hospital Discharge Survey and National Survey of Ambulatory Surgery that arthrodesis procedures have increased 146% with outpatient arthrodeses increasing by 415%. Subtalar joint arthrodesis is a commonly used procedure in foot and ankle surgery for various pathologic conditions. Grice and colleagues[2] were the first to describe an isolated subtalar arthrodesis in 1952. Generally, subtalar arthrodeses are performed in conjunction with other procedures but they can be done in isolation. The rates of union for subtalar joint arthrodesis have been generally positive, with more recent literature showing cohorts achieving 100% union.[3] The purpose of a subtalar arthrodesis is typically pain relief, realignment

[a] The Reconstruction Institute, The Bellevue Hospital, 1400 West Main Street, Bellevue, OH 44811, USA; [b] Progressive Feet, 611 South Carlin Springs Road, Suite 508, Arlington, VA 22204, USA
* Corresponding author.
E-mail address: PeterDHighlander@gmail.com

Clin Podiatr Med Surg 40 (2023) 633–648
https://doi.org/10.1016/j.cpm.2023.05.007
0891-8422/23/© 2023 Elsevier Inc. All rights reserved.

for deformity correction, and functional improvement of the rearfoot.[4] Although subtalar arthrodesis is typically done in conjunction with other procedures, there seems to be an increase in isolated approaches likely secondary to shorter operation times and preservation of hindfoot motion.[5] According to Astion and colleagues,[5] fusion of the subtalar joint limited motion of the talonavicular joint by 74% and of the calcaneocuboid joint by 44%. Nonunion remains one of the most concerning challenges foot and ankle surgeons face when dealing with subtalar arthrodeses.[6] There have been publications demonstrating increased rate of nonunions in patients with smoking history, diabetes, neuropathy, trauma, infection, obesity, revision surgery, devascularized bone, and previous ankle fusion.[7,8] Surgeons have made various attempts to optimize outcomes despite risk factors, focusing on changes in technique, construct, and augmentation with bone grafts.

PERTINENT ANATOMY

The subtalar joint is defined as the 3 facet joints between the plantar talus and the dorsal calcaneus. These facets are known as the anterior, middle, and posterior facets, with the largest being posterior. Between these 2 bones is the interosseous talocalcaneal ligament as well as the artery of the tarsal canal, which anastomoses with the artery of the sinus tarsi. The medial aspect of this joint is known at the tarsal canal, whereas the lateral-most aspect is known as the sinus tarsi. These facets create the subtalar joint, which moves about a single joint axis for triplane motion of pronation and supination. A normal ratio of pronation to supination is considered to be 2:1. This joint is understandably very important in ambulation, as it controls a majority of shock absorption through pronation and rigidity for push-off through supination.[9] This plays a role in surgical technique, focusing on strong compression across the middle and posterior facets and avoiding exuberant amounts of hardware across the talar neck to lessen chances of vascular compromise.

INDICATIONS

Indications for isolated subtalar joint arthrodesis include primary arthritis, posttraumatic arthritis, inflammatory arthritis, subtalar coalition, posterior tibial tendon dysfunction (PTTD), and other hindfoot deformities. Osteoarthritis and inflammatory arthritis require subtalar arthrodesis when bracing and medication have failed to control symptoms and pain. Subtalar arthrodesis is often performed in conjunction with other procedures, such as tibiotalocalcaneal arthrodesis, double versus triple arthrodesis, as well as a variety of osteotomies and ancillary procedures, including gastrocnemius recession and bone grafting. Posttraumatic arthritis is a very well-documented sequela known to occur following intra-articular calcaneal fractures. Calcaneal fractures in and of themselves can be quite a challenge to reduce and fixate, but certain complications have been documented to happen owing to inadequate fixation and/or other patient factors.[10] Failure modes of reduction can increase the occurrence of posttraumatic arthritis involving the following: loss of calcaneal height, hindfoot varus, lateral wall widening, or impingement. Revision to subtalar arthrodesis can be more challenging owing to these factors as well as existing hardware, leading the surgeon to consider grafting and/or corrective osteotomies. Although a subtalar coalition can technically occur between any of the 3 facets, the middle facet is the most common.[11] Subtalar coalitions are known to have a bimodal distribution affecting ages 12 to 16 years and again later in adulthood.[12] Subtalar coalitions typically require an arthrodesis, as resection alone has poor outcomes owing to secondary arthritic changes, especially in an older population. Progressive deformity associated with

PTTD follows a predictable pattern as described by Johnson and Strom.[13] In later stages of PTTD, the hindfoot has developed arthritic changes and has become a rigid deformity. Arthrodesis of the affected hindfoot joints is indicated in late-stage PPTD. Similarly, arthrodesis is indicated in arthritic varus hindfoot deformities.

SURGICAL TECHNIQUE

Approach and positioning for revision subtalar arthrodesis are often dependent on the presence or absence of deformity, such as loss of calcaneal height and/or previous incisions/scars, retained hardware, and soft tissue quality. Typically, the patient is positioned in a supine position with an ipsilateral hip bump to control external rotation. Incisional approaches to be considered in a supine position include lateral sinus tarsi, posterolateral, and medial. Generally speaking, laterally based approaches allow for better access and visualization of the joint, but a medial approach allows the surgeon to gain direct access to the articulating surfaces (described in detail in Chapter 5). The advent of an arthroscopic approach has also become more popularized in recent years.[14] The authors tend to favor a lateral sinus tarsi incision for revisions unless loss of calcaneal height is a concern, in which case a posterior approach is more likely with prone positioning. If there is a need for removal of hardware as one may expect with revisions, one may need to position and place the incision or incisions accordingly, including anterior/posterior or lateral extensile.

A combination of sharp and blunt dissection should be used to dissect down through superficial and deep fascia until the extensor retinaculum and extensor digitorum brevis are encountered, at which point sharp reflection superiorly should take place. Carefully locate the sinus tarsi and lateral process of the talus through manipulation. In revision cases, this is often difficult to assess because of previous fixation and potential pseudarthrosis. The surgeons recommend the use of fluoroscopic guidance with a Kirschner wire or osteotome to help attain visualization. If there is a partial union, an osteotomy or saw may be useful here. Once the subtalar joint is exposed, a pin distractor, such as a Hintermann, or a lamina spreader can be used to enhance intra-articular visualization and access, thus ensuring adequate joint preparation. In a primary arthrodesis, the goal is to prepare both sides of the joint to bleeding bone that can be well opposed with proper fixation. This can be performed using several manual instruments, such as rongeurs, osteotomes, curettes, and power tools, such as burrs and drills. Joint preparation is the key to success in revision cases as well but can be more demanding owing to the presence of fibrous tissue, nonunion, and pseudoarthrosis. All nonviable tissue needs to be properly resected before preparing the bony surfaces. Following joint preparation, bone grafting should be considered. This consideration should help the surgeon decide between various allografts, autografts, or a combination. As discussed later, autograft seems to be preferred, which is harvested from the proximal or distal tibial metaphysis. If large bone defects are present or significant deformity correction is required, a structural graft may be needed. Structural autograft from the pelvis may be considered but is associated with higher morbidity. Structural allograft is another option however may be cost prohibitive and has higher rates of nonunion if there is a large defect.[15,16] Other options for deformity correction or large osseous defects are the utilization of three-dimensional (3D)-printed titanium cages.[17] The authors prefer to use metallic porous 3D-printed wedges and cages with deformity correction or with large defects. These customizable 3D-printed implants provide long-lasting structural support and inherent stability owing to surface roughness and can be packed with bone graft or biologics. These 3D-printed implants are scaffolds, which are osteoconductive, and in the authors' experience, are more reliable for defects greater than 2 cm. Once the desired position is achieved, guide wires for desired size screws are placed. There are a multitude of different orientations or size configurations of subtalar joint arthrodesis. For primary subtalar fusions, the authors prefer 2 to 3 large partially threaded headless cannulated screws. In revision cases, fixation and stability may be more difficult to achieve owing to bone quality, previously placed hardware, and voids. The authors have found intra-medullary nails that provide dynamic compression to be the most reliable.

In cases with secondary deformity, such as loss of calcaneal height and talar dorsi-flexion and/or significant varus leading to impingement, the authors prefer prone positioning with a central-posterior incision placement. This incision allows for access to the posterior subtalar joint, preparation of the joint, and placement of graft for restoration of alignment. A similar fixation construct as above is used unless the goal is to maintain distraction and alignment; then 2 fully threaded screws are used to prevent graft collapse.[18] The posterior approach allows for Achilles tendon lengthening to be easily performed, which is often helpful in restoring sagittal plane alignment of the talus and calcaneus and allows for adequate distraction to be maintained. The authors often approach the subtalar joint directly through the Achilles tendon using a central incision.[19] A Z-lengthening of the Achilles tendon is performed, and the proximal/distal aspects are reflected, which enhance visualization of the posterior facet. The Achilles tendon is repaired in a lengthened position before final closure.

CONSIDERATIONS/CURRENT EVIDENCE
Fixation Options

Fixation options to be considered consist of large solid, cannulated screws, or intra-medullary nailing. There is general debate on the number of screws (one, two, three) and orientation of the screws (divergent or parallel vs anterior to posterior or posterior to anterior) in terms of which fixation method is superior. There is even some debate into the size of screws typically ranging between 6.5 and 8.0 mm in screw size. Current evidence supports that the delta configuration as discussed by Hungerer and colleagues[20] has the strongest biomechanical stability. Hungerer and colleagues[20] demonstrated in their study by comparing parallel, counter-parallel, and delta configurations, that the delta configuration had the greatest biomechanical stiffness with the lowest degree of deflection in cadaveric models. This study also demonstrated no difference when comparing 6.5- versus 8.0-mm sized screws as well as no difference using cannulated versus solid screws. Another biomechanical study performed by Chuckpaiwong and colleagues[21] challenged several different screw constructs and compared compression, torsional stiffness, and least amount of joint rotation. The constructs they compared included single screw in the talar dome, single screw in the talar neck, double parallel screws, and double diverging screws. According to this study, double-diverging screws was the best construct in all parameters measured. A single 7.0-mm screw construct directed across the posterior facet as discussed by Haskell and colleagues[22] demonstrated 98% fusion rate (99/101) with an average time to fusion being 12.3 weeks. Interestingly, Haskell and colleagues[22] demonstrated increased time to fusion with a prior ankle fusion, but revision subtalar fusion did not affect time to fusion. Each of the patients in this 101 patient cohort did receive autograft from the sinus tarsi and anterior process of the calcaneus. Davies and colleagues[4] also demonstrated great results using a single-screw construct with a single 7.0-mm partially threaded cancellous screw for fixation in both primary and revisional subtalar arthrodesis. Davies and colleagues[4] were able to demonstrate a union rate of 95% in 95 primary isolated subtalar arthrodeses. Decarbo and colleagues[23] published a study comparing 1- versus 2-screw fixation for their subtalar arthrodesis demonstrating no significant difference. Bofelli and colleagues[24] in a 15-patient study demonstrated the efficacy of using their unique 2-screw construct. This unique screw construct includes a typical compression screw across the posterior facet from posterior to anterior but also includes a second screw from the plantar lateral aspect of the anterior calcaneus into the talar head or neck, which is considered a stability screw. Their study had a 100% union rate.[24]

More recently, Wirth and colleagues[25] in 2020 published their article on comparing a 2- versus 3-screw construct for subtalar joint arthrodesis. Their article demonstrated a statistically significant increased rate of nonunion and increased rate of revision surgeries in the 2-screw construct compared with the 3-screw construct in 113 patients. The investigators also concluded that diabetes, a high body mass index (>30), and having a prior ankle fusion surgery increased the need for revision arthrodesis. Similarly, a study by Jones and colleagues[26] demonstrated a decrease in time to fusion as well as a decreased rate of nonunion in the 3-screw construct (N = 28) compared with the 2-screw construct (N = 26) in a cohort of 54 patients. Specifically, the 3-screw construct group had zero nonunions, whereas the 2-screw construct group had a nonunion rate of 26.9%. There does not seem to be a definitive answer in the literature when it comes to screw constructs, but it is the authors' opinion that 2 partially threaded headless screws spanning the subtalar joint in a divergent pattern are sufficient in most cases with primary arthrodesis.

More recently, subtalar joint-specific implants and intramedullary nails have been introduced to be used for primary or revision arthrodesis. When considering revision options, the authors believe fixation should be more robust by increasing the size or number of fixation points that differ in placement from that used in primary fusion surgery. Intramedullary nailing with cancellous autograft is the authors' method of choice when considering revision options. Intramedullary nailing provides effective stable fixation with minimally invasive placement.[27,28] Furthermore, devices with the ability to provide static and dynamic compression enhance stability and may improve outcomes. Dynamic compression provided by internal NiTiNoL (Nickel Titanium-Navel Ordinance Laboratory) technology provides 2 to 4 mm of active compression in addition to manual static front-loading compression. This is particularly important if aforementioned patient risk factors contribute to potential nonunion.[29]

Bone Graft

The use of bone grafts is to provide osteogenesis, osteoinduction, osteoconduction, and/or structural support. The formation and resorption of bone carried out at the subtalar level are continuous, and interruption or insufficiency of any of the metabolic pathways involved may lead to poor outcomes in patients undergoing osseous surgery, including arthrodesis. There are advantages and disadvantages between different bone grafts, whether autogenous or allograft. Not all bone grafts will have the same properties; therefore, surgeons should consider the patient demographics and comorbidities as well as the specific indication to aid in identifying the ideal graft for that particular situation.[30–32] An overview comparing various bone graft options is provided in **Table 1**.

Successful subtalar joint arthrodesis using autograft and screw fixation has been reported for nearly half a century.[33] Although autograft in many regards remains the gold standard for osseous procedures because it possesses all qualities necessary while maintaining histocompatibility, quantity and quality of autografts are limited and may be dependent on patient demographics and comorbidities.[30,32] Harvesting

Table 1
Properties, advantages, disadvantages, and examples of bone graft options

	Source	Properties	Advantages	Disadvantages	Examples
Autograft	• Obtained from the patient • Corticocancellous vs cancellous • Multiple harvest sites to consider	• Osteoinductive • Osteoconductive • Osteogenetic • Structural support (corticocancellous sources only)	• Traditionally considered gold standard • No risk of disease transmission • Structural & nonstructural options • Cancellous sources provide superior osteoconductive, osteoinductive, & osteogenic properties • Corticocancellous sources provide structural support • Vascularized options enhance osteogenic properties & provide structural support • Various harvesting techniques & instrumentation exist • No direct cost associated	• Donor site morbidity is site dependent • Limited quantity • Quality is dependent on patient demographics & comorbidities • Added surgical time • Increased blood loss	*Corticocancellous* • Iliac crest • Calcaneus *Cancellous* • Tibial metaphysis (proximal vs distal) • Calcaneus • Bone marrow aspirate
Allograft	Cadaveric donors	• Osteoconductive • Variable osteoinduction	• Unlimited quantity • Structural & nonstructural options • Minimal added surgical time • Fresh cadaveric grafts & DBM maintain some osteoinductive properties • Lower cost compared with synthetic substitutes & BMPs	• Integration not as effective as autograft • Possible host-disease transmission	• Fresh structural cadaveric • Frozen structural cadaveric • Freeze-dried cancellous chips • DBM

Synthetic substitutes	Bioengineered/synthetic ceramics	• Structural • Osteoconductive	• Unlimited quantity • Provides structural support and scaffolding to allow osteointegration • Primarily used to fill bone defects to provide structural support	• Variable integration & resorption rates • Minor osteoconductive properties • Cost typically higher than allografts	• Calcium sulfate • Calcium phosphate • Tricalcium phosphate • Coralline hydroxyapatite • Magnesium phosphate
Bone morphogenetic proteins	Bioengineered/synthetic	• Osteoinductive • Osteogenetic	• Naturally found in bones & used by multiple organs for maintenance & development • Promotes guided tissue regeneration	• Markedly most expensive option • Nonstructural • Limited FDA approval • Limited indications • Wide spectrum of adverse outcomes reported • Theoretical carcinogenesis	• rhBMP-2 • rhBMP-7 • rhBMP-11 • rhPDGF

autograft also carries a higher risk of morbidity, which is dependent on harvest site location and quantity of graft harvested compared with allografts. Morbidity is often associated with the harvest site location, the type of graft harvested, and quantity of graft harvested. Fundamentally, cortical-cancellous provides structural support while being less metabolically active than purely cancellous sources. Cancellous autograft is nonstructural but much more cellular, and therefore, incorporates into the donor site more readily.[30,34] For example, Attia and colleagues[35] demonstrated a morbidity rate of 6.8% when harvesting from the proximal tibial metaphysis (Gerdy tubercle), distal tibia metaphysis, or calcaneus, which is less than half of the known morbidity rate of harvesting a cortical-cancellous iliac crest graft. Furthermore, the investigators reported, of the 3 lower-extremity sites, calcaneal grafts were associated with significantly more complications, including chronic pain, fractures, and sural neuritis as compared with grafts obtained from the tibia.

There may be situations when allograft should be used in place of autograft. There is no perceived limit of allograft available and there is no association with increased operative time or harvest site morbidity. Cadaveric allografts are available in cancellous and cortical forms, or as demineralized bone matrix (DBM). Allografts possess osteoconductive properties, and DBM-processing methods allow retention of osteoinductive properties; however, allografts have no osteogenic properties therefore do not incorporate as readily. Allografts also carry the potential for disease transmission.[35,36]

Clinical comparison of autograft and allografts used for subtalar joint arthrodesis has been retrospectively reported. Easley and colleagues[7] reported results of 184 subtalar joint arthrodeses in 174 patients, which included 28 revision cases. All cases were fixated with 1 or 2 screws, whereas 145 of 184 cases received either cancellous autograft (n = 94), structural autograft (n = 29), cancellous allograft (n = 17), or structural allograft (n = 5). The investigators reported an 86% union rate from primary cases and 71% union rate in revision cases. Of note, 3 out of the 5 structural allografts in this study went on to nonunion, but because of limited data, they could not demonstrate a significant relationship between the type of bone graft and the rate of union or the time to union.

In a large retrospective study, Davies and colleagues[4] performed 95 isolated subtalar arthrodeses where autograft was used in 92 of the patients. The investigators reported a 95% union rate, whereas 4 patients required revision for nonunion. The autograft used included structural iliac crest graft for restoration of calcaneal height in posttraumatic arthritis cases, as well as cancellous autograft from the tibia, fibula, or calcaneus.[4] Joveniaux and colleagues[37] reported a series of 28 isolated subtalar arthrodeses with an average of 56-month follow-up. The investigators found a 100% union rate in both 16 cases with iliac crest and 10 cases with allograft. They fixated each subtalar joint using 1 to 2 staples and demonstrated 100% union rate. This study suggests that outcomes of primary subtalar joint fusion may not necessarily be influenced by graft source.

Allogeneic bone grafts are known to be relatively safe; however, reports on union rates have been mixed. In a retrospective review, Scranton[38] compared 12 open, isolated subtalar arthrodeses using iliac crest autogenous bone graft versus 5 arthroscopic arthrodeses using bone morphogenic protein (BMP). In this study, Scranton[38] demonstrated no significant difference when comparing union rates or postoperative complications. This study did demonstrate a longer tourniquet time by 5 minutes on average in the arthroscopic group compared with the open group, but the length of hospital stay on average was higher in the open group. Michelson and Curl,[39] in a prospective study, compared autograft from the iliac crest with

DBM in 55 patients undergoing either isolated subtalar arthrodesis or triple arthrodesis; 18 patients received autograft, whereas 37 received DBM. They demonstrated no difference between cohorts when it came to union rates. Both autograft and allogeneic options can be used when providing structural grafts for deformity correction when performing subtalar joint arthrodesis.

Synthetic bone substitutes have been shown to have a positive patient-safety profile and relatively similar fusion rates to autograft and allograft and are increasingly cost-effective. There is seemingly a plethora of options when it comes to considering synthetic grafts, including calcium sulfate, tricalcium phosphate, biphasic calcium phosphate, hydroxyapatite, bioglass, magnesium, and silicate calcium phosphate. In a published cohort of 17 patients, Fusco and colleagues[40] demonstrated only 70% fusion rate at 12 weeks using biphasic calcium phosphate. This study by Fusco and colleagues[40] used biphasic calcium phosphate for both revisions and primary fusions. In a larger study performed by Shah and colleagues,[41] 135 subtalar arthrodeses were performed, of which 82 received tricalcium phosphate mixed with bone marrow aspirate, 8 received DBM, 2 received iliac crest autograft, one received allograft cancellous chips, and the rest did not receive any graft. They demonstrated a union rate of 88 without graft and 83 with grafting, suggesting these synthetic grafts may not be needed.

BMPs are naturally found growth factors that promote and guide tissue-specific growth. Literature has shown the following BMPs have proven osteogenic properties; BMP2, BMP6, BMP7, and BMP11.[42] Various BMPs are involved in the different stages of bone healing, which can prove beneficial in achieving arthrodesis.[43] Various preclinical reports have shown increased levels of different BMPs during stages of auto-induction, formation of progenitor cells, increasing bone turnover, and promoting remodeling.[43,44] Autograft proves superior in BMP concentrations given its native source; however, this is variable based on the host and may not be currently upregulated by the host. Through the utilization of recombinant DNA technology, there are commercially available BMPs available to add to surgical sites. These are inherently osteogenic and osteoinductive; however, they provide no structural integrity. Cost-effectiveness is of concern but can prove useful in the compromised host. Kanakaris and colleagues[45] achieved a healing rate of 90% in 19 joint fusions (ankle, subtalar, talonavicular, pubic, and sacroiliac) with the use of rhBMP-7 (recombinant bone-morphogenetic proteins). There is further literature using rhBMP-2 in various spinal fusion reports but limited research focusing on lower-extremity arthrodesis procedures and the isolated use of BMPs as adjunctive graft.

In cases of posttraumatic deformity, such as decreased calcaneal height, traditionally structural cadaveric allografts or tricortical iliac crest graft have been used. With the advent of 3D-printing technology, customized, patient-specific porous metallic wedges and cages are available and are particularly useful for severe osseous deficits and/or significant deformity. The macroscopic porous quality allows for nonstructural graft or bone substitute to be packed into the implant. The microscopic porous structure mimics that of cancellous bone, which historically plays the primary role of osteoinduction. However, traditional methods of harvesting cancellous bone yield graft with poor handling characteristics, creating poor graft retention, and therefore, allograft and substitutes are used. The senior author has developed a method for efficient graft harvest that then allows for the solid and liquid portions of the graft to be separated using the Hensler Bone Press (Hensler Surgical Technologies, Wilmington, NC, USA). The patented methodology improves handling characteristics of the cancellous autograft, allowing it to be easily packed into porous 3D-printed implants while enhancing graft retention. The use of specialized bone graft harvesters do add direct cost but decreases operative time. The direct cost of using the Hensler Bone Press is $550 to $700, which is far less than competing devices that do not improve handling characteristics. The authors prefer to harvest cancellous graft from the proximal or distal tibia owing to lower morbidity compared with the calcaneus.[35] In addition, it is the authors' experience that a larger quantity of graft can be obtained from the tibia. It should be emphasized that the authors' preferences are currently anecdotal, as there are no published comparative reports at the time of writing this article. In an ovine cortical and cancellous model, Kelly and colleagues[46] demonstrated a linear relationship between porosity of 3D implants and mechanical properties but a parabolic relationship between porosity and pushout strength. This study demonstrated the highest pushout strength of the porous titanium gyroid implants at a 4-week and 12-week time point was 60% porosity implants. However, there has been a significant increase in the foot and ankle literature to the efficacy and ability of patient-specific 3D-printed porous cages for osseous deficits.[47–49]

Case Reports

Patient 1 is a 52-year-old man who presented with hindfoot pain. The patient underwent a previous subtalar joint arthrodesis with a two-screw construct that ultimately failed, including broken hardware (**Fig. 1**). Upon revision, most of the hardware was removed; the nonunion was resected, and both sides of the joint were reprepared. Tibial autograft was harvested and placed within the fusion site. The area was fixated and compressed with an intramedullary nail. After a period of non-weight-bearing, the patient demonstrated union at 8 weeks on radiographs and confirmed union at 10 weeks on computed tomographic (CT) scan. The patient went on to heal successfully and returned to ambulation without pain and use of an ASO brace (**Fig. 2**). Approach and intraoperative approach of a similar case requiring a custom-printed metallic wedge are depicted in **Fig. 3**.

Patient 2 is a 37-year-old man who presented with hindfoot pain. The patient underwent a previous subtalar joint arthrodesis with a 2-screw construct that ultimately failed with a frank hypertrophic nonunion (**Fig. 4**). Upon revision, the hardware was removed; the nonunion was resected, and both sides of the joint were reprepared. Tibial autograft was harvested and placed within the fusion site. The area was fixated and compressed with an intramedullary nail (Envois Lewisville, TX). Serial radiographs demonstrated union at 6 weeks, confirmed on CT scan at 10 weeks. The patient went on to heal successfully and returned to ambulation without pain and in regular shoes (**Fig. 5**). Approach and intraoperative approach of a similar case requiring a custom-printed metallic wedge are depicted in **Fig. 6**.

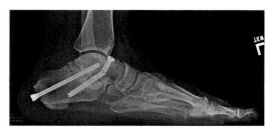

Fig. 1. Patient 1: preoperative radiograph at time of presentation.

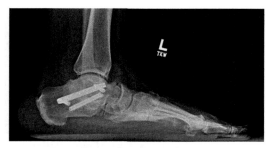

Fig. 2. Patient 1: postoperative radiograph at time of union.

DISCUSSION

Subtalar joint arthrodesis is a commonly used procedure for numerous pathologic conditions. Although rarely performed in isolation, they generally have a high rate of union with limited complications. However, patient factors, including cause of pathologic

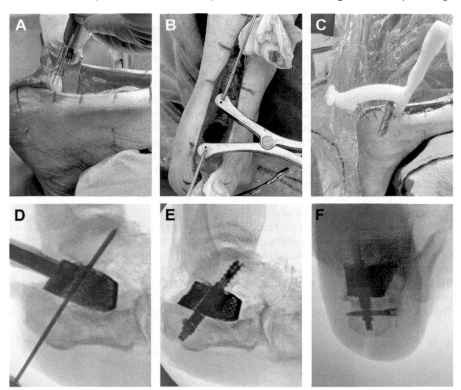

Fig. 3. (*A–F*) Patient initially presented as a 65-year-old woman with past medical history of diabetic neuropathy and rheumatoid arthritis with a malunion of her intra-articular calcaneal fracture. Because of the loss of height, the senior author elected to restore alignment using a custom 3D-printed titanium cage(Retor3d, Durham NC). (*A*) A custom 3D-printed cut guide with temporary wire fixation. (*B*) The resection of calcaneus. (*C, D*) One of the trials/insertion of a 3D-printed custom cage implant with precision pin placement using this guide. (*E, F*) Placement of calcaneal intramedullary nail(Envois Lewisville, TX) across the 3D implant for isolated revision subtalar joint arthrodesis.

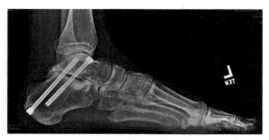

Fig. 4. Patient 2: preoperative radiograph at time of presentation.

condition, can contribute to an increased rate of nonunion. When nonunion or malunion is to be addressed, the authors recommend the following considerations.

It is imperative to identify patient factors that may have contributed to nonunion, which then should be corrected or optimized before considering revision surgery. Surgical technique, fixation selection and augmentation, and use of bone graft to the revision are imperative to increase chances of union. Multiple approaches exist, and selection is dependent on prior incision and hardware placement, as well as presence of deformity and/or osseous deficit. Joint preparation is paramount for obtaining fusion and often can be more time consuming as compared with primary cases. With numerous fixation options discussed in literature, having a robust and rigid fixation construction is critical to revision arthrodesis. Fixation for revision cases should be more robust than that used in the previous failed procedure, which can be challenging depending on previously placed hardware that requires removal, which yields additional osseous compromise. The authors recommend a similar approach to the "superconstruct" methodology as described by Sammarco[50] when considering fixation. The surgeon should consider using more points of fixation (ie, increasing the number of screws), larger fixation options as well as altering the orientation of the fixation construct. The authors have found intramedullary fixation that has the ability to provide postoperative dynamic compression in addition to traditional manual static compression achieved intraoperatively.

Although the literature has no stout consensus on type or use of bone graft, autograft remains superior with uncompromised success particularly with revision arthrodesis. The authors use a specialized technique to harvest a significant amount of nonstructural bone from the tibial metaphysis (proximal or distal). With the use of the Hensler Bone Press, this can be performed with minimal increase in operative times, increased graft handling characteristics with improved quality of autograft. The authors strongly recommend harvesting tibial bone graft with revision arthrodesis.

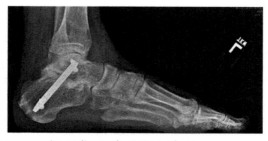

Fig. 5. Patient 2: postoperative radiograph at time of union.

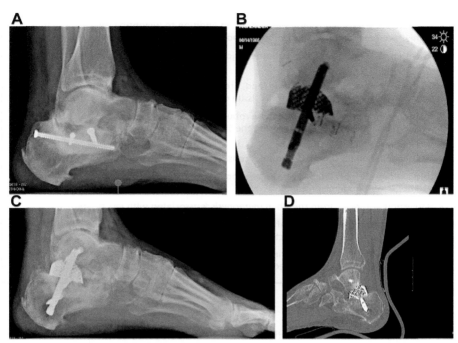

Fig. 6. (*A–D*) Patient was a 54-year-old man who initially presented 4 years following an open reduction and internal fixation of an intra-articular calcaneal fracture from an outside hospital. (*A*) In-office preoperative consult lateral projection showing depressed posterior facet with arthritic changes in the subtalar joint. (*B*) Intraoperative positioning and placement of 3D custom cage and intramedullary nail. (*C, D*) At his 3-month postoperative office visit demonstrating satisfactory alignment, no hardware failure, and osseous ingrowth within the cage.

As discussed above, the authors present 2 cases with frank nonunion of the subtalar joint. In both cases, intramedullary nailing and harvesting of tibial autograft were performed yielding success results.

SUMMARY

Although subtalar joint arthrodesis is rare, care should be taken to optimize the patient and approach when performing revisional subtalar joint arthrodesis. Given that isolated arthrodesis is not known to commonly fail, this signifies the importance of identifying factors that may be contributory to failure and addressing them upon revisional surgery.

CLINICS CARE POINTS

- Subtalar joint arthrodesis may be performed in isolation or in conjunction with adjacent joint arthrodesis, osteotomies, and other ancillary procedures.
- Revision subtalar joint arthrodesis is associated with lower union rates and increased time to union as compared with primary subtalar joint arthrodesis.
- Infection must be ruled out or treated if subtalar joint nonunion is encountered.

- Preoperative computed tomographic scans, in addition to weight-bearing radiographs, are highly recommended to assess deformity, bone quality, and presence of osseous defects
- As with primary subtalar joint arthrodesis, joint preparation is paramount but can be more time consuming.
- Multiple approaches can be used and are determined by the presence of deformity, previously placed hardware, and soft tissue quality.
- Fixation during revision should be more robust than primary cases, which can be achieved by increasing point of fixation, increasing the size of fixation, and altering the orientation of fixation.
- Intramedullary nails should be strongly considered for revision subtalar joint arthrodesis.
- Using autograft is preferable but can be supplemented with allografts, synthetic substitutes, and bone morphogenic proteins.
- Harvesting autograft from the tibial metaphysis is associated with less morbidity,
- Utilization of specialized autograft harvesting instrumentation may decrease operative time while enhancing handling characteristics,
- Patient-specific 3-dimensional-printed titanium alloy implants should be considered when deformity and/or substantial osseous defects are encountered.

DISCLOSURE

R.J. Lerch, DPM and Amar Gulati, DPM have no disclosures or conflicts. Peter Highlander, DPM is a consultant for Restor3d, Inc (Durham, NC) and Hensler Surgical Technologies, LC (Wilmington, NC).

REFERENCES

1. Best MJ, Buller LT, Miranda A. National trends in foot and ankle arthrodesis: 17-year analysis of the national survey of ambulatory surgery and national hospital discharge survey. J Foot Ankle Surg 2015;54(6):1037–41.
2. Grice DS. An extra-articular arthrodesis of the subastragalar joint for correction of paralytic flat feet in children. J Bone Joint Surg 1952;34-A:927–40.
3. Lee KB, Park CH, Seon JK, et al. Arthroscopic subtalar arthrodesis using a posterior 2-portal approach in the prone position. Arthroscopy 2010;26(2):230–8.
4. Davies MB, Rosenfeld PF, Stavrou P, et al. A comprehensive review of subtalar arthrodesis. Foot Ankle Int 2007;28:295–7.
5. Astion DJ, Deland JT, Otis JC, et al. Motion of the hindfoot after simulated arthrodesis. J Bone Joint Surg Am 1997;79(2):241–6.
6. Chraim M, Recheis C, Alrabai H, et al. Midterm outcomes of subtalar joint revision arthrodesis. Foot Ankle Intl 2021;42(7):824–32.
7. Easley ME, Trnka HJ, Schon LC, et al. Isolated subtalar arthrodesis. J Bone Joint Surg Am 2000;82(5):613–24.
8. Zura R, Mehta S, Della Rocca GJ, Steen RG. Biological Risk Factors for Nonunion of Bone Fracture. JBJS Rev 2016;4(1):e5. https://doi.org/10.2106/JBJS.RVW.O.00008.
9. Rockar P. The subtalar joint: anatomy and joint motion. J Orthop Sports Phys Ther 1995;21(6):361–72.
10. Buckley R, Tough S, McCormack R, et al. Operative compared with nonoperative treatment of displaced intra-articular calcaneal fractures: a prospective, randomized, controlled multicenter trial. J Bone Joint Surg Am 2002;84(10):1733–44.

11. Kulik S, Clanton T. Tarsal coalition. Foot Ankle Int 1996;17(5):286–96.
12. Schwartz J, Kihm C, Camasta C. Subtalar joint distraction arthrodesis to correct calcaneal valgus in pediatric patients with tarsal coalition: a case series. J Foot Ankle Surg 2015;54(6):1151–7.
13. Johnson KA, Strom DE. Tibialis posterior tendon dysfunction. Clin Orthop Relat Res 1989;239:196–206.
14. Bannerjee S, Gupta A, Elhence A, et al. Arthroscopic subtalar arthrodesis as a treatment strategy for subtalar arthritis: a systematic review. J Foot Ankle Surg 2021;60(5):1023–8.
15. Lee MS, Tallerico V. Distraction arthrodesis of the subtalar joint using allogeneic bone graft: a review of 15 cases. J Foot Ankle Surg 2010;49(4):369–74.
16. Myerson M, Quill GE. Late complications of fractures of the calcaneus. J Bone Joint Surg 1993;75(A):331–41.
17. Parry E, Catanzariti AR. Use of three-dimensional titanium trusses for arthrodesis procedures in foot and ankle surgery: a retrospective case series. J Foot Ankle Surg 2021;60(4):824–33.
18. Pollard J, Schuberth J. Posterior bone block distraction arthrodesis of subtalar joint: a review of 22 cases. J Foot Ankle Surg 2008;47(3):191–8.
19. Highlander P, Greenhagen RM. Wound complications with posterior midline and posterior medial leg incisions: a systematic review. Foot Ankle Spec 2011;4(6):361–9.
20. Hungerer S, Eberle S, Lochner S, et al. Biomechanical evaluation of subtalar fusion: the influence of screw configuration and placement. J Foot Ankle Surg 2013;52:177–83.
21. Chuckpaiwong B, Easley ME, Glisson RR. Screw placement in subtalar arthrodesis: a biomechanical study. Foot Ankle Int 2009;30:133–41.
22. Haskell A, Pfeiff C, Mann R. Subtalar joint arthrodesis using a single lag screw. Foot Ankle Int 2004;25(11):774–7.
23. DeCarbo WT, Berlet GC, Hyer CF, et al. Single-screw fixation for subtalar joint fusion does not increase nonunion rate. Foot Ankle Spec 2010;3:164.
24. Boffeli TJ, Reinking RR. A 2-screw fixation technique for subtalar joint fusion: a retrospective case series introducing a novel 2-screw fixation construct with operative pearls. J Foot Ankle Surg 2012;51:734–8.
25. Wirth SH, Viehofer A, Fritz Y, et al. How many screws are necessary for subtalar fusion? A retrospective study. J Foot Ankle Surg 2020;26(6):699–702.
26. Jones JM, Vacketta VG, Philp FH, Catanzariti AR. Radiographic Outcomes of Isolated Subtalar Joint Arthrodesis With Varying Fixation Technique. J Foot Ankle Surg 2022;61(5):938–43.
27. Goldzak MP, Simon P, Mittlmeier T, et al. Primary stability of an intramedullary calcaneal nail and an angular stable calcaneal plate in a biomechanical testing model of intraarticular calcaneal fracture. Injury 2014;45:S49–53.
28. Reinhardt S, Martin H, Ulmar B, et al. Interlocking nailing in intraarticular calcaneal fractures: a biomechanical study of two different interlocking nails vs. an interlocking plate. Foot Ankle Int 2016;37(8):891–7.
29. Bernasconi A, Iorio P, Ghani Y, et al. Use of intramedullary locking nail for displaced intraarticular fractures of the calcaneus: what is the evidence? Arch Orthop Trauma Surg 2022;142:1911–22.
30. Cho W, Nessim A, Gartenberg A, et al. Racial differences in iliac crest cancellous bone composition: implications for preoperative planning in spinal fusion procedures. Clin Spine Surg 2022;35(3):E400–4.

31. Fillingham Y, Jacobs J. Bone grafts and their substitutes. J Bone Joint Surg 2016; 98-B:6–9.
32. Guerado E, Fuerstenberg CH. What bone graft substitutes should we use in post-traumatic spinal fusion. Injury 2011;42(2):S64–71.
33. Dennyson WG, Fulford GE. Subtalar arthrodesis by cancellous grafts and metallic internal fixation. J Bone Joint Surg Brit 1976;58-B4:507–10.
34. Walsh WR, Pelletier MH, Wang T, et al. Does implantation site influence bone ingrowth into 3D-printed porous implants? Spine J 2019;19(11):1885–98.
35. Attia AK, Mahmoud K, ElSweify K, et al. Donor site morbidity of calcaneal, distal tibial, and proximal tibial cancellous bone autografts in foot and ankle surgery. A systematic review and meta-analysis of 2296 bone grafts. J Foot Ankle Surg 2022;28(6):680–90.
36. Roberts TT, Rosenbaum AJ. Bone grafts, bone substitutes and orthobiologics: the bridge between basic science and clinical advancements in fracture healing. Organogenesis 2012;8:114–24.
37. Joveniaux P, Harisboure A, Ohl X, et al. Long-term results of in situ subtalar arthrodesis. Int Orthop 2010;34(8):1199–205.
38. Scranton PE Jr. Comparison of open isolated subtalar arthrodesis with autogenous bone graft versus outpatient arthroscopic subtalar arthrodesis using injectable bone morphogenic protein-enhanced graft. Foot Ankle Int 1999;20(3):162–5.
39. Michelson JD, Curl LA. Use of demineralized bone matrix in hindfoot arthrodesis. Clin Orthop Relat Res 1996;325:203–8.
40. Fusco T, Sage K, Rush S, et al. Arthrodesis of the subtalar joint using a novel biphasic calcium phosphate bone graft. FASTRC 2022;2(1).
41. Shah A, Naranje S, Araoye I, et al. Role of bone grafts and bone graft substitutes in isolated subtalar joint arthrodesis. Acta Ortop Bras 2017;25(5):183–7.
42. Dumic-Cole I, Peric M, Kucko L, et al. Bone morphogenetic proteins in fracture repair. Int Orthop 2018;42:2619–26.
43. Vukicevic S, Oppermann H, Verbanac D, et al. The clinical use of bone morphogenetic proteins (BMPs) revisited: a novel BMP6 biocompatible carrier device Osteogrow for bone healing. Int Orthop 2014;38:635–47.
44. van Baardewijk LJ, van der Ende J, Lissenberg-Thunnissen S, et al. Circulating bone morphogenetic protein levels and delayed fracture healing. Int Orthop 2013;37:523–7.
45. Kanakaris N, Mallina R, Calori GM, et al. Use of bone morphogenetic proteins in arthrodesis: clinical results. Injury 2009;53:562–6.
46. Kelly CN, Wang T, Crowley J, et al. High-strength, porous additively manufactured implants with optimized mechanical osseointegration. Biomaterials 2021; 276:121206. https://doi.org/10.1016/j.biomaterials.2021.121206.
47. Lachman JR, Adams SB. Tibiotalocalcaneal arthrodesis for severe talar avascular necrosis. Foot Ankle Clin 2019;24(1):143–61.
48. Adams SB, Danilkowicz RM. Talonavicular joint-sparing 3D printed navicular replacement for osteonecrosis of the navicular. Foot Ankle Int 2021;42(9): 1197–204.
49. Abar B, Kwon N, Allen NB, et al. Outcomes of surgical reconstruction using custom 3D-printed porous titanium implants for critical-sized bone defects of the foot and ankle. Foot Ankle Int 2022;43(6):750–61.
50. Sammarco VJ. Super constructs in the treatment of Charcot foot deformity: plantar plating, locked plating and axial screw fixation. Foot Ankle Clin N Am 2009;14:393–407.

Triple Arthrodesis
How to Manage Failures, Malunion, and Nonunion

Jacob M. Perkins, DPM, AACFAS[a],*,
Vincent G. Vacketta, DPM, AACFAS[a], Mark A. Prissel, DPM, FACFAS[b]

KEYWORDS

- Malunion • Triple arthrodesis • Revision surgery • Deformity correction

KEY POINTS

- Malunion and/or nonunion are the typical complications of triple arthrodesis.
- A thorough understanding of the normal biomechanics and rectus positioning of the foot and ankle are required to adequately treat revision cases.
- Patient comorbidities, index deformity, and index procedure information are important in determining why a nonunion occurred.
- Earlier hardware may prevent adequate fixation and require more extensive solutions.
- Nonunions can be superimposed into malunion complications.

INTRODUCTION

The triple arthrodesis procedure has an established and effective history in treating a host of foot and ankle pathologic conditions due to the drastic corrective ability. Ryerson published the classic technique in 1923, referencing and modifying an earlier technique described by Hoke who did not utilize or mention calcaneocuboid fusion.[1,2] Although Ryerson primarily used the procedure for hindfoot stabilization of polio patients, the indications have progressively expanded to other hindfoot deformities such as that in talipes equinovarus, end-stage pes planus, and for severe hindfoot arthritic deformities.[3] There is a significant amount of research validating triple arthrodesis, and although a surgical "success" can have different criteria among

[a] Orthopedic Foot and Ankle Center Advanced Foot and Ankle Reconstruction Fellowship, 350 W. Wilson Bridge Road, Street. 200, Worthington, OH 43085, USA; [b] Advanced Foot and Ankle Reconstruction, Orthopedic Foot and Ankle Center, 350 W. Wilson Bridge Road, Street. 200, Worthington, OH 43085, USA
* Corresponding author.
E-mail address: jacobmichaelperkins@gmail.com

Clin Podiatr Med Surg 40 (2023) 649–668
https://doi.org/10.1016/j.cpm.2023.05.008
0891-8422/23/© 2023 Elsevier Inc. All rights reserved.
podiatric.theclinics.com

physicians and publications, it has been reported approximately 85% to 95% of patients have successful procedures.[4,5]

What accounts for the 5% to 15% of failures most commonly involves nonunion and malunion, which intuitively correlates to the surface area of multiple fusion sites and the complicated weight-bearing biomechanics of the hindfoot solidified into a rigid construct. The frequency of nonunion has changed as techniques have become more refined over the years; however, rates of malunion involving overcorrection or undercorrection have remained similar.[5]

Although the history and efficacy of triple arthrodesis is well documented, revisional treatment and management is not as published. The index procedure is already very technically challenging, so the revision of complications can create an extremely difficult task for the foot and ankle surgeon. It is important to characterize malunion failures versus nonunion failures despite their potential interconnectedness in order to fully identify causes of the outcome because the superimposition of one can blur the importance of the other.

NONUNION

Nonunion within triple arthrodesis has varying rates in the literature ranging from 0% to 29%.[5,6] Postulated reasons for nonunion are many, and they need to be considered especially in the revision arthrodesis patient. Comorbidities, drug use, nutritional deficiencies, potential infection, and fixation constructs are just a few examples of the considerations when evaluating a revision arthrodesis candidate. Moreover, as referenced earlier, a nonunion in combination with malalignment will only further complicate the surgical treatment plan. It is important to note the patient clinically because there are instances where a radiographic nonunion is asymptomatic and not of biomechanical concern. Preoperative computed tomography (CT) scans to confirm and to elucidate the characteristics of nonunion are necessary.

A 2018 retrospective study by Klassen and colleagues evaluated 152 patients who underwent triple arthrodesis from 2007 to 2013. Their primary outcome was to find the joint of triple arthrodesis most common to nonunion, with secondary measures to correlate nonunion to patient demographics and joint preparation techniques. They found the nonunion rates of TNJ, CCJ, and STJ at 20.4%, 17.2%, and 8.9%, respectively. Of significance, they found patients who underwent fish scaling rather than resection or curettage alone had associated lower nonunion rates.[6] This finding correlates to a 2009 histological study by Johnson and colleagues where they found curettage alone did not adequately resect the calcified layer of articular cartilage, which could potentially contribute to nonunion.[7] This intuitively directs the revisional surgeon to take particular care to evaluate intraoperatively the earlier arthrodesis surfaces.

For the studies that have lower reported percentages of nonunion, one study by Bednarz and colleagues reported a 97% fusion rate. They attribute potentially a reasoning for this rate was the use of iliac crest bone graft in 89% of their patients; however, of note, there was only 1 patient out of 57 that was a smoker.[8,9] Although it is unclear in this study if the union rate is attributed more toward the use of bone graft versus the patient population, it is important to make this distinction because one of the most significant risk factors for nonunion that is also one of the most modifiable is smoking. In a recent 2021 study by Allport and colleagues, they found a profound relative risk ratio of 5.81 in relation to nonunion in smokers versus nonsmokers.[10] To have such a severely high risk in a revision arthrodesis patient, it is extremely important to consider this factor in an already at-risk patient population. Patient education, selection, and medical stabilization is key.

Incision placement to remove earlier hardware must be considered, especially if concomitant deformity correction must take place. When accessing the nonunion joint, a similar fixation might not be feasible due to the inherent nature of the primary fixation method and whatever osseous implication it may have had, such as large diameter screw holes adjacent to cortical surfaces. This may not only exclude prior fixation but also require more fixation than the index procedure to make a stable construct. Bone graft in these scenarios is wise; however, a conundrum must be addressed: if patient factors/comorbidities contributed to the initial nonunion (ie diabetes), allograft rather than autograft can be considered. If addressing additional deformity correction, structural graft versus impaction bone grafting can further be used.[11]

CLINICS CARE POINTS: NONUNION

- In the preoperative workup, consider additional testing related to comorbidities or other variables that can be medically stabilized to support fusion
- When considering incision placement, care must be taken to have exposure to prior hardware removal if indicated
- Fixation that initially failed has decreased viable bone purchase, use adjacent fixation that may need to be supported by additional fixation to make a stable construct
- Bone graft to support arthrodesis is normally best taken from the patient; however, consider allograft in a poor host

MALUNION

Rates of malunion vary within the literature and seem to correlate with more severe deformity at the index procedure. Overall rates have been cited near 6%, with equinovarus being the most common orientation.[5] A 1997 study by Haddad and colleagues reported their series of revisional triple arthrodesis having, in descending frequency, equinovarus with or without rocker bottom, varus hindfoot, valgus hindfoot, and simple rocker bottom residual deformity. In their discussion, they revealed 3 technical reasons for malunion including surgeon's inadequate understanding of degree of deformity, recurring deformity drivers such as in progressive neuromuscular diseases, and third, where surgeon appreciation of deformity and correction is present, however, is unable to surgically achieve adequate reduction.[12] The literature has traditionally represented and categorized the type of malunion into varus/valgus, dorsiflexion/plantarflexion, or abduction/adduction.[5,12,13] This intuitively suits this concept as the corrective revision procedure is dictated by the type of malunion.

General concepts for reduction are similar to primary procedures in that rearfoot deformity is normally corrected first, which will allow the true forefoot position to elucidate and can subsequently be corrected as indicated. For the revision case specifically, a preoperative CT scan is imperative for the evaluation of solid fusion among the tri-joint complex. The goals of reduction are to achieve an ankle at neutral to slight plantarflexion ($0°–5°$), hindfoot at neutral to slightly valgus ($0°–5°$), and forefoot with mild abduction ($10°–15°$). If reduction is not adequate from joint alignment alone, then adjunct procedures may need to be performed, such as calcaneal osteotomy as one example. Moreover, it is imperative that any residual forefoot varus is accounted for, sometimes requiring an ancillary Cotton osteotomy or plantarflexory first tarsometatarsal arthrodesis. As referenced before, Haddad and colleagues notably published an algorithm that follows hindfoot to forefoot correction while addressing specific apices of deformity, and this algorithm is referenced frequently in the literature.[5,12] In 33 patients, they identified the plane in which the apex of the deformity occurred and surgically addressed proximally either with closing wedge or insertion of bone block. In 29 feet, they achieved arthrodesis with this methodology with a significant reduction in pain scores.[12] In 2001, Bibbo and colleagues published a study with similar categorization of deformity as Haddad; however, they had more specific techniques with different combinations of rear, hind, and forefoot deformities.[13] Toolan, later in 2004, published an article investigating the novel use of biplanar, opening-closing osteotomies that addressed valgus hindfoot, forefoot abduction rocker bottom deformities in the severely undercorrected triple. Discussed further below, Toolan acknowledges the earlier-cited literature; however, he suggests his technique could prevent the extensive osteotomies and concurrent foot shortening associated with those earlier techniques.[14]

Many of the concepts in these publications are still widely referenced and used to this day and are discussed more in detail below. Of note, the established literature specifically addressing the correction of the malunited triple arthrodesis is sparse, and these concepts have remained essentially unchanged in the literature for the past 20 years. Furthermore, it is important to recognize that these deformities may be multiplanar and have multiple adjunct procedures needed or with use of biplanar wedges and through and through derotational osteotomies.[5] Often in these complex cases, the soft tissue components can be underappreciated but may still require correction including tendon transfers/lengthening of the peroneals and stabilization/reconstruction of the lateral (varus malunion) and or medial (valgus malunion) ankle ligaments.

Hindfoot Varus Malunion

The malunion subcategories of varus and valgus types seem to be the most commonly encountered in the literature and have been cited to occur approximately 3% frequency. In relation to failure of the primary arthrodesis, they have also been cited in older literature as accounting for 11% of failures. Varus hindfoot malunion alone is relatively uncommon in isolation, and normally has a forefoot component to it. This is normally attributed to deformity within the subtalar joint fusion. The general concept to understand is that proximal varus essentially contributes to lateral column overload because it begins to exceed inherent compensatory eversion. In isolation and in deformities where only mild-moderate correction is needed, a closing wedge lateral displacement calcaneal osteotomy has been described.[5,12,13] Over translation laterally is a potential complication of this procedure, which can lead to iatrogenic tarsal tunnel.[15,16] It is important to note that forefoot supinatus can be elucidated by preoperative submetatarsal 5 callus, which suggests compounded deformity and need for further correction.

More severe hindfoot varus malunions occur when, in addition to varus malalignment from the subtalar joint, the midtarsal joint is also fused with varus malposition. Patients will walk on the lateral column of their foot and have noted callosities to the fifth metatarsal head and base.[13] Haddad and colleagues suggested an additional closing wedge osteotomy through the STJ fusion site; however, intuitively this requires a transverse osteotomy through the midtarsal fusion block or else the subtalar wedge cannot be appositioned.[12] A particular scenario that Bibbo and colleagues recommended in this context is if the STJ varus matches the MTJ varus, in which both can be potentially corrected via Dwyer osteotomy through the calcaneus. Furthermore, in a category of the most severe varus combination that Bibbo and colleagues describes and rearfoot and hindfoot varus with ankle varus, a supramalleolar osteotomy is recommended. Depending on the chronicity and intraoperative findings, lateral ligament procedures with or without deltoid recessions will help in further reduction.[13]

Hindfoot Valgus Malunion

A hindfoot valgus malunion in triple arthrodesis parallels many symptoms seen in flatfoot deformities. Subfibular impingement, fibular stress fracture, and potential tarsal tunnel symptoms are possibilities in this general architecture.[5,13] More long-term, eventual deltoid ligament failure from medial stress and subsequent ankle valgus and arthritis has been described as a predictable sequela.[17-19] Certainly if the primary triple arthrodesis was done to address a severe flatfoot indication, residual deformity is a possibility. This is sometimes seen in our experience as an arthritic valgus hindfoot that was fused in situ without deformity correction, possibly because surgical goals at the time of primary surgery concentrated on relieving more clinically acute arthritis. Another explanation is presented in an article by Rush where they describe excessive lateral subtalar debridement in combination with inadequate debridement of the anterior and middle facets of the subtalar joint position the rearfoot in a valgus bias.[17] Typically, residual flatfoot deformity is tolerated more than overcorrection into varus; however, if still clinically significant symptoms persist, revisional arthrodesis may be the best option. Although undercorrection is most common, this is not to say an overcorrected varus deformity could not present as a valgus malunion.

Treatment referenced commonly in the literature of both Bibbo and colleagues and Haddad and colleagues describe sufficient treatment with medial displacement calcaneal osteotomy.[5,12,13] More recent literature has suggested that calcaneal osteotomies can only correct small degrees of valgus and that further procedures may be indicated.[17,20] One of these publications by Shi and colleagues in 2017 describe lateral column lengthening via calcaneocuboid distraction arthrodesis using approximately 0.6 to 1.0 cm tricortical graft. Additionally touted benefits of this procedure are that they correct multiple planes that can all be affected by the malunited triple, including transverse plane abnormalities. Although the article vaguely describes criteria as to when a lateral column lengthening distraction arthrodesis would benefit, other authors discussing in this context describe talar head uncovering of greater than 40%.[21]

There are some patients fused with severe hindfoot valgus that would not be sufficiently treated by calcaneal osteotomy and concomitantly have additional midfoot abduction, creating a rocker bottom deformity. Toolan has described the treatment of this scenario, in which a closing wedge of the medial talar neck is used in combination with a lateral opening wedge of the cuboid/calcaneus.[14] The osteotomy is through-and-through the talus to the lateral column, and the harvested medial wedge is placed, after osseous shaping, into the gap created on the lateral column. There were 5 patients described in the publication, and each had an improvement of foot alignment, clinical ratings, and patient satisfaction.

Calcaneal Height

Within the context of malunion arises a shortened calcaneus within the subtalar portion of the triple arthrodesis, commonly a depressed posterior facet. This can bias the talus into increased inclination and cause the ankle joint to proceed into a pseudo impingement. To restore normal alignment a calcaneal osteotomy with distraction interpositional bone graft, such as tricortical iliac crest, has been described.[13]

CLINICS CARE POINTS: MALUNION

- Preoperatively measure severity of malunion deformities and plan for the osteotomies appropriately, undercorrection or overcorrection on a secondary surgery will leave even less options in the future
- Take multiple view intraoperative fluoroscopic images, compare to preoperative images, and visibly evaluate foot alignment with each chosen procedure
- Length is addressed via addition or removal of bone, rotation is determined from the angle of the osteotomy or the wedge applied, and three-dimensional understanding of which is required at what level can be supported by CT scan

---

LONG-TERM COMPLICATIONS: SECONDARY OSTEOARTHRITIS

A question that arises within the context of this article subject is what constitutes surgical "failure." Certainly, malreduction and malunion to a certain degree causing intolerable pain and function in the acute postoperative setting would suffice; however, it should be noted that even in surgical "success" populations, it has been described that the increase in pressures and strains on adjacent joints can accelerate their arthritic progression. In a 2007 cadaveric study by Suckel and colleagues, they found an increase in ankle joint peak pressures following triple arthrodesis in comparison to isolated talonavicular arthrodesis.[22] A 2014 study by Ebalard and colleagues had a multicenter retrospective study of degenerative secondary arthritis in patients who underwent triple arthrodesis versus isolated joint fusion with a minimum of 10-year follow-up. They found that the rate of secondary osteoarthritis determined radiographically in the tibiotalar joint at the final visit was as high as 73%.[23] The authors of this study note that there was no statistical significance of secondary tibiotalar arthritis and patient symptoms; however, there were significantly higher pain scores at the final follow-up of patients than at the 12-month follow-up, which they postulate as a relation to secondary arthritic formation. Regardless, before index surgical procedure, the patient should be appropriately counseled on potential arthritic change at adjacent joints over time that may require further surgical intervention.

CASE REPORTS
Case #1

We present a case from our institution that illustrates this concept with just one of the joints fused. **Figs. 1–12** present the preoperative, perioperative, and postoperative relevant images of the case. A 68-year-old woman presented with complaints of inability to walk secondary to lateral ankle pain. Formerly an active walker, she had a long reported history of flat foot deformity that has failed bracing and wanted to pursue a more definitive solution. Her radiographs are presented below. Clinical and radiographic findings included moderate subtalar arthritis, navicular-cuneiform sag, posterior tibial tendon dysfunction (PTT) deficiency, moderate forefoot flexibility, fibula stress fracture, and noted moderate talo-navicular uncoverage. Her

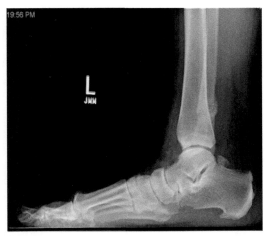

Fig. 1. Preoperative images of index pathology.

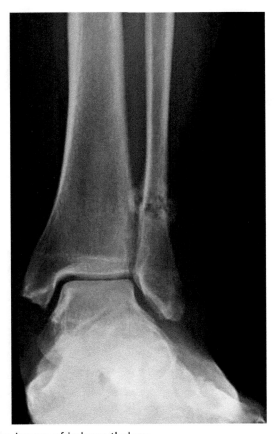

Fig. 2. Preoperative images of index pathology.

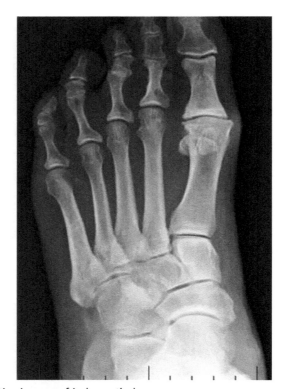

Fig. 3. Preoperative images of index pathology.

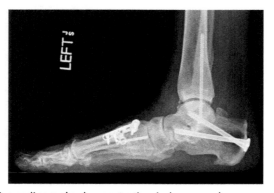

Fig. 4. Postoperative radiographs demonstrating index procedure.

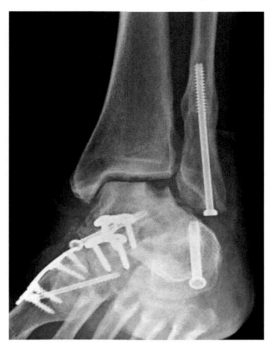

Fig. 5. Clinical radiographs 9 months status after index procedure. Left is non–weight-bearing, right is weight-bearing. This demonstrates the malunited rearfoot positioning effect on the ankle joint.

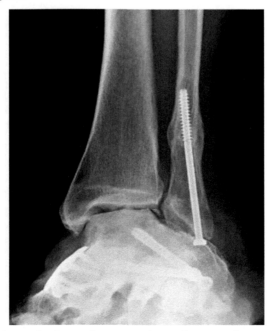

Fig. 6. Clinical radiographs 9 months status after index procedure. Left is non–weight-bearing, right is weight-bearing. This demonstrates the malunited rearfoot positioning effect on the ankle joint.

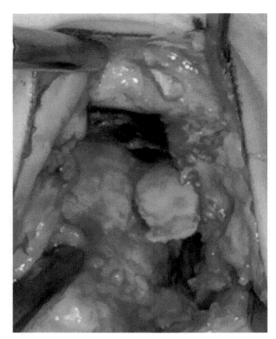

Fig. 7. Intraoperative view of ankle joint demonstrating articular collapse.

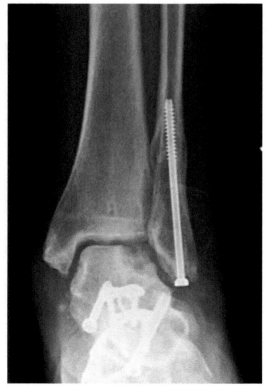

Fig. 8. Postoperative varus deformity correction procedure.

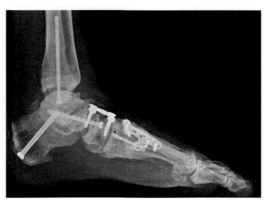

Fig. 9. Postoperative varus deformity correction procedure.

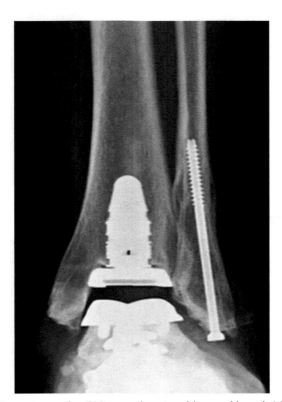

Fig. 10. Immediate postoperative TAR procedure to address ankle arthritis sequela.

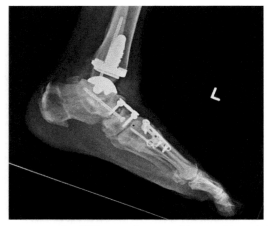

Fig. 11. Immediate postoperative TAR procedure to address ankle arthritis sequela.

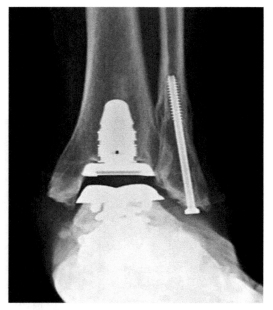

Fig. 12. One-year postoperative TAR.

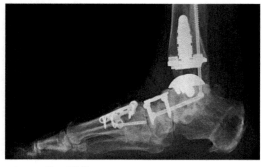

Fig. 13. One-year postoperative TAR.

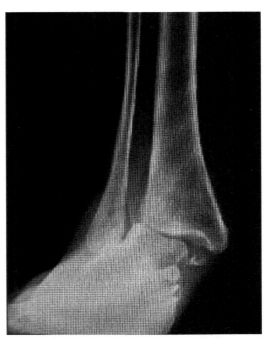

Fig. 14. Preoperative imaging of acute ankle fracture predisposed from valgus malunion of triple arthrodesis.

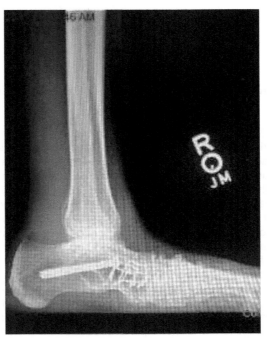

Fig. 15. Preoperative imaging of acute ankle fracture predisposed from valgus malunion of triple arthrodesis.

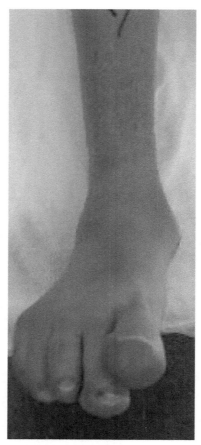

Fig. 16. Clinical presentation demonstrating medial malleolar soft tissue injury.

initial operative (OR) intervention included a subtalar fusion, and flexor digitorum longus transfer (FDL) transfer, a first tarsal metatarsal (TMT) fusion, and an open reduction internal fixation (ORIF) of the fibula. She underwent an uneventful postoperative course until 9 months later she presented with worsening, severe ankle pain. Non–weight-bearing and weight-bearing radiographs demonstrate ankle valgus compensation for a malunited and aligned rearfoot arthrodesis. Specifically, residual forefoot varus that was not corrected during index surgery. The patient returned to the operating room for revision of the forefoot varus via talonavicular (TN) fusion and ankle arthrotomy. The varus was successfully corrected and the patient further went on to an ankle replacement 6 months later to address the ankle arthritis that was now deformity corrected. The patient healed successfully and 1-year postoperative radiographs are displayed. Although only one of the joints in the context of this article was initially fused in this patient, it was still enough to cause malunion of the hindfoot positioning leading to ankle arthritis. An article by Hyer and colleagues found that triple arthrodesis had a 3.64 higher chance of later valgus ankle arthritis than double arthrodesis, which further illustrates that although this case does not have a triple, the concept in this setting is applicable.[24]

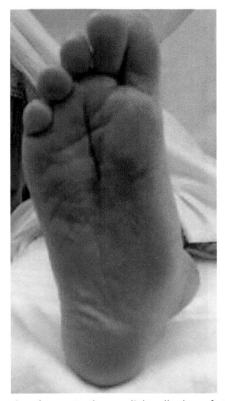

Fig. 17. Clinical presentation demonstrating medial malleolar soft tissue injury.

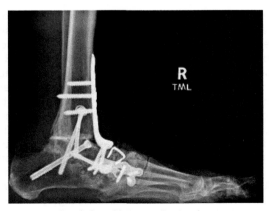

Fig. 18. A 3-month postoperative deformity correction/acute treatment procedure involving ankle arthrodesis and midfoot rotational osteotomy.

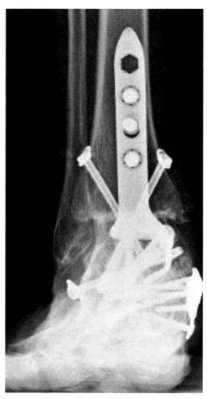

Fig. 19. A 3-month postoperative deformity correction/acute treatment procedure involving ankle arthrodesis and midfoot rotational osteotomy.

Case #2

Another case from our institution is presented. **Figs. 13–22** illustrate clinical and radiographic preoperative, perioperative, and postoperative findings. An 85-year-old healthy woman with a past surgical history of triple arthrodesis more than 2 decades earlier presented to the clinic with complaints of right foot/ankle pain after having a "missed a step" 6 weeks before presentation. Initial ER XR was negative, and the patient stated she did not pursue further treatment because the foot alignment appeared normal to her. Clinically she had pain to the medial aspect of the ankle with associated soft tissue defect on the verge of ulceration. Radiographic findings included malunited triple arthrodesis with severe hindfoot valgus with sagittal collapse, midfoot and ankle degenerative joint disease (DJD), and forefoot varus associated with a more acute unstable trimalleolar fracture. Surgically she underwent an ankle fusion with a derotational midfoot osteotomy to correct the valgus deformity. Uneventful postoperative course until 10 months where she experienced a tibial stress fracture due to the ankle fusion fixation construct and severe rigidity of her rearfoot. She did not want further surgery and was conservatively managed with an ankle foot orthosis (AFO) brace that subsequently healed her stress fracture and she remains ambulatory without soft tissue or alignment

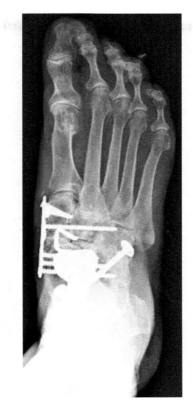

Fig. 20. A 3-month postoperative deformity correction/acute treatment procedure involving ankle arthrodesis and midfoot rotational osteotomy.

concerns. This illustrates the potential acute and chronic stressors of a malunited triple arthrodesis causing a potentially predisposed valgus moment, which made a "misstep" a trimalleolar fracture compounded by chronic ankle arthritis sequela.

Case 1: Treatment of Ankle Arthritis Sequelae Status Post Malunited Hindfoot Fusion

Figures for case 1 courtesy of Dr Gregory Berlet, MD. Orthopedic Foot and Ankle Center, Columbus, OH.

Case 2: Treatment of an Acute Low Energy Trauma Predisposed by Valgus Malunion

Figures for case 2 are courtesy of Dr Mark Prissel, coauthor of article and attending at Orthopedic Foot and Ankle Center, Columbus, OH.

DISCLOSURE

No funding was received for this publication and there are no conflicts of interest.

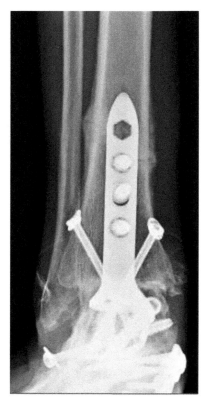

Fig. 21. A 13-month postoperative radiographs demonstrating healing stress fracture of tibia.

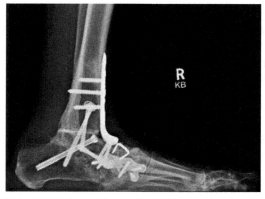

Fig. 22. A 13-month postoperative radiographs demonstrating healing stress fracture of tibia.

REFERENCES

1. Brand RA. Arthrodesing operations on the feet. Clin Orthop Relat Res 2008; 466:5–14.
2. Hoke M. An operation for stabilizing paralytic feet. Amer J Orthop Surg 1921;3: 494–507.
3. Bennett GL, Graham CE, Mauldin DM. Triple arthrodesis in adults. Foot Ankle 1991;12(3):138–43.
4. Saltzman CL, Fehrle MJ, Cooper RR, et al. Triple arthrodesis: twenty-five and forty-four-year average follow-up of the same patients. J Bone Joint Surg Am 1999;81(10):1391–402.
5. Seybold JD. Management of the malunited triple arthrodesis. Foot Ankle Clin 2017;22(3):625–36.
6. Klassen LJ, Shi E, Weinraub GM, et al. Comparative nonunion rates in triple arthrodesis. J Foot Ankle Surg 2018;57(6):1154–6.
7. Johnson JT, Schuberth JM, Thornton SD, et al. Joint curettage arthrodesis technique in the foot: a histological analysis. J Foot Ankle Surg 2009;48(5):558–64.
8. Bednarz PA, Monroe MT, Manoli A 2nd. Triple arthrodesis in adults using rigid internal fixation: an assessment of outcome. Foot Ankle Int 1999;20(6):356–63.
9. Wilson FC Jr, Fay GF, Lamotte P, et al. Triple Arthrodesis. A Study of the factors affecting fusion after three hundred and one procedures. J Bone Joint Surg Am 1965;47:340–8.
10. Allport J, Ramaskandhan J, Siddique MS. Nonunion rates in hind- and midfoot arthrodesis in current, ex-, and nonsmokers. Foot Ankle Int 2021;42(5):582–8.
11. Burns PR, Powers NS. Revisional triple and pantalar arthrodesis. In: Zgonis T, Roukis TS, editors. Revisional and reconstructive surgery of the foot and ankle. 1st edition. Pennsylvania Furnace, PA: Lippincott Williams & Wilkins; 2023. p. 186–210.
12. Haddad SL, Myerson MS, Pell RF, et al. Clinical and radiographic outcome of revision surgery for failed triple arthrodesis. Foot Ankle Int 1997;18(8):489–99.
13. Bibbo C, Anderson RB, Davis WH. Complications of midfoot and hindfoot arthrodesis. Clin Orthop Relat Res 2001;391:45–58.
14. Toolan BC. Revision of failed triple arthrodesis with an opening-closing wedge osteotomy of the midfoot. Foot Ankle Int 2004;25(7):456–61.
15. Bruce BG, Bariteau JT, Evangelista PE, et al. The effect of medial and lateral calcaneal osteotomies on the tarsal tunnel. Foot Ankle Int 2014;35(4):383–8.
16. Southwell RB, Sherman FC. Triple arthrodesis: a long-term study with force plate analysis. Foot Ankle 1981;2(1):15–24.
17. Rush SM. Reconstructive options for failed flatfoot surgery. Clin Podiatr Med Surg 2007;24(4):779–88.
18. Song SJ, Lee S, O'Malley MJ, et al. Deltoid ligament strain after correction of acquired flat foot deformity by triple arthrodesis. Foot Ankle Int 2000;21(7):573–7.
19. Resnick RB, Jahss MH, Choeueka J, et al. Deltoid ligament forces after tibialis posterior tendon rupture: effects of triple arthrodesis and calcaneal displacement osteotomies. Foot Ankle Int 1995;16(1):14–20.
20. Shi E, Weinraub GM. Lateral column lengthening for revision triple and double arthrodesis and severe end-stage flatfoot deformity. J Foot Ankle Surg 2019; 58(3):577–80.
21. Hunt KJ, Farmer RP. The undercorrected flatfoot reconstruction. Foot Ankle Clin 2017;22(3):613–24.

22. Suckel A, Muller O, Herberts T, et al. Talonavicular arthrodesis or triple arthrodesis: peak pressure in the adjacent joints measured in 8 cadaver specimens. Acta Orthop 2007;78(5):592–7.

23. Ebalard M, Le Henaff G, Sigonney G, et al. Risk of osteoarthritis secondary to partial or total arthrodesis of the subtalar and midtarsal joints after a minimum follow-up of 10 years. Orthop Traumatol Surg Res 2014;100(4 Suppl):S231–7.

24. Hyer CF, Galli MM, Scott RT, et al. Ankle valgus after hindfoot arthrodesis: a radiographic and chart comparison of the medial double and triple arthrodeses. J Foot Ankle Surg 2014;53(1):55–8.

The Ankle Joint
Non-Operative Updates in Ankle Arthritis, Are Biologics Working?

Kyle S. Peterson, DPM, FACFAS[a],*, Vincent Vacketta, DPM, AACFAS[b], Amber Kavanagh, DPM, AACFAS[c]

KEYWORDS

- Ankle arthritis • Nonsurgical • Conservative • Corticosteroids • Platelet-rich plasma
- Amion • Hyaluronic acid

KEY POINTS

- Ankle arthritis most frequently develops after traumatic injury and is diagnosed using a combination of patient history, physical examination, and imaging.
- Options for the conservative management of symptoms include the use of physical therapy, bracing, and injectables.
- The use of injectable corticosteroids, hyaluronic acid, platelet-rich plasma, and amniotic tissue-derived products have all shown promising results in the literature for the treatment of ankle arthritis.

INTRODUCTION

Ankle arthritis is a debilitating musculoskeletal condition that leads to pain and impaired mobility. While it is difficult to assess the incidence of ankle arthritis, literature suggests it affects approximately 2% to 5% of people to varying degrees.[1] When compared to other joints such as the knee and hip, primary osteoarthritis (OA) is less commonly found in the ankle joint due to better joint congruency for optimal loading and stiffer cartilage with less response to inflammatory cytokines.[1–3] There are a handful of causes for arthritis in the ankle such as OA, trauma, inflammation related to gout or rheumatoid, avascular necrosis, lower extremity deformity, and hemophilia. The majority of ankle arthritis, however, is post-traumatic in nature, with rates of 60% to 80% reported in the literature.[4,5] Injury to the ankle resulting from fracture, or even severe sprains can accelerate the rate of cartilage degeneration leading to painful symptoms in younger patients, thus necessitating treatment earlier in life.

[a] Suburban Orthopaedics, 1110 West Schick Road, Bartlett, IL 60103, USA; [b] Orthopedic Foot and Ankle Center Fellowship, 350 West Wilson Bridge Road, Suite. 200, Worthington, OH 43085, USA; [c] Hinsdale Orthopaedics (IBJI) Foot and Ankle Fellowship, 951 Essington Road, Joliet, IL 60435, USA
* Corresponding author.
E-mail address: kyle.s.pete@gmail.com

Clin Podiatr Med Surg 40 (2023) 669–680
https://doi.org/10.1016/j.cpm.2023.05.009
0891-8422/23/© 2023 Elsevier Inc. All rights reserved.

CLINICAL PRESENTATION

There are a handful of signs and symptoms associated with ankle arthritis. Early clinical symptoms involve pain with joint range of motion. This pain usually begins gradually and only persists in activities with higher loading. As the joint continues to degenerate, pain can even occur at rest. Patients relate that certain movements can exaggerate their pain level. For example, uphill activity often aggravates joint pathology at the anterior ankle, while pain on a downhill motion is related to disease at the posterior ankle.[6] Swelling and stiffness are also common patient complaints. On physical exam, decreased range of motion noted at the ankle joint is encountered frequently. This can be due to joint incongruity, cartilage loss, osteophyte formation, intra-articular fragments, as well as contractures of the capsule and peri-articular ligaments. Joint crepitus on attempted range of motion and effusion can also be observed. The pain on palpation along the anterior ankle joint or in the ankle gutters can be due to osteophytes or joint inflammation.[7]

DIAGNOSTIC IMAGING AND STAGING

Imaging is essential for the diagnosis of ankle arthritis. Radiographs are useful in assessing joint space narrowing, subchondral sclerosis, bony erosion, osteophytes, and adjacent osteopenia.[8] An example of this is shown in **Fig. 1**. While plain film radiographs reveals some joint changes, advanced imaging such as computed tomography (CT) scan and magnetic resonance imaging (MRI) can better demonstrate joint degeneration as they are more sensitive. CT allows for a more specific illustration of bony erosions. Some of the findings that present on CT scan in these patients include better evaluation of bone quality and density, sclerosis, subchondral cyst formation, smaller bony erosions, osseous deformity, coalitions, joint ankylosis, smaller osteophytes, and joint congruency.[8] These changes appreciated on CT are shown in **Fig. 2**. MRI is often termed the gold standard in evaluating for early joint changes in ankle arthritis. This is due to its

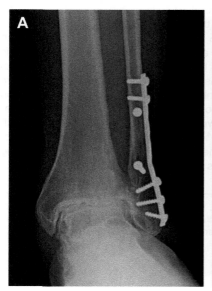
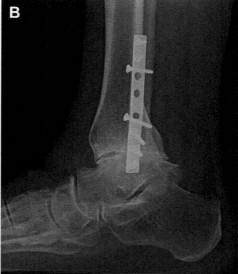

Fig. 1. (*A*) AP and (*B*) lateral ankle radiographs showing severe joint space narrowing and subchondral sclerosis in a patient with posttraumatic ankle arthritis.

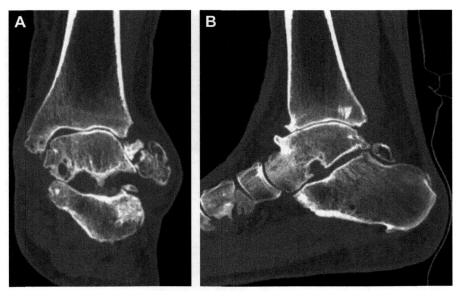

Fig. 2. (*A*) Coronal and (*B*) sagittal ankle views on CT scan demonstrating narrowed joint space, sclerosis, cyst formation, anterior joint osteophytes, and joint incongruence.

ability to visualize synovitis, often seen in inflammatory arthritides. MRI can also reveal bone erosions and associated bone marrow edema, cartilage thinning, osteochondral defects, avascular necrosis, and adjacent ligament damage.[5,8] An example of this is demonstrated in **Fig. 3**. Dohn and colleagues compared plain film radiographs to advanced imaging and found that CT and MRI were superior in diagnosing bony erosions.[9] Ultrasound (US) is a less common modality that can also be used to visualize early joint changes in arthritis. These include soft tissue changes such as synovitis, joint effusion, adjacent soft tissue edema, and osteophyte formation.[8]

There are several staging classifications used to separate ankle arthritis based on observations from plain film radiographs. The two most commonly used are the Giannini classification and the Takakura classification system.[10,11] These are demonstrated in **Tables 1** and **2**. These classification systems are useful in diagnosing the degree of degenerative changes in order to utilize the proper treatment protocol.

NON-OPERATIVE THERAPEUTIC OPTIONS

Non-operative treatment strategies for ankle arthritis focus on joint immobilization and a plethora of injectable options aimed at reducing inflammation and slowing the rate of cartilage degeneration in the joint. These conservative options are important to highlight as they are the first line of therapy in most patients before considering surgery, and alone may be able to provide the desired pain relief. In other cases, surgical treatment is not an option due to patient comorbidities or socioeconomic factors. Conservative care, therefore, is the only choice available in these cases to allow people to return to a functional life.

PHYSICAL THERAPY

Physical therapy can be used in some patients in the early stages of ankle arthritis to help with the management of symptoms. Therapists have a number of modalities

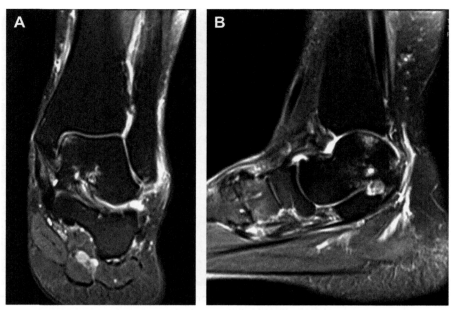

Fig. 3. (A) Coronal and (B) sagittal ankle views on MRI revealing anterior joint effusion, decreased joint space, bone marrow edema, and osteochondral defect.

including thermotherapy, ultrasound, and transcutaneous electrical nerve stimulation that help with managing symptoms associated with arthritis. In treating inflammatory arthritides, it has been shown that low-level laser therapy in combination with these other modalities has been of clinical benefit to patients.[5,12] In developing a plan for therapy, it is important to categorize the joint into either inflammatory and non-inflammatory, or stable and unstable. This can help guide the proper therapeutic protocol to prevent further irritation to the joint. In an inflammatory state, treatment is focused around anti-inflammatory medications, cold therapy, and limiting mobility. In a non-inflamed joint, therapy programs usually focus on adjacent muscle strengthening and joint mobilization in both the hindfoot as well as the ankle. The same differentiation in therapy is true for stable and unstable joints. In an unstable joint, the goal is to brace the ankle while allowing for some mobilization exercises and strengthening activities. If stable, the ankle can be mobilized, however, it is key to utilize orthotics or shoe modifications in conjunction to help restore the native biomechanics of the foot to the ankle.[13]

Table 1	
Giannini et al ankle osteoarthritis classification system	
Stage	**Radiographic Signs**
Stage 0	Normal joint or subchondral sclerosis
Stage 1	Presence of osteophytes without joint space narrowing
Stage 2	Joint space narrowing, with or without osteophytes
Stage 3	Subtotal or total disappearance or deformation of joint space

Table 2
Takakura et al ankle osteoarthritis classification system

Stage	Radiographic Signs
Stage 1	No joint-space narrowing, but early sclerosis and osteophyte formation
Stage 2	Narrowing of the joint space medially
Stage 3	Obliteration of the joint space with subchondral bone contact medially
Stage 4	Obliteration of the whole joint space with complete bone contact

BRACING AND SHOE MODIFICATIONS

Controlling the biomechanics of the foot and ankle with bracing or shoe modifications is important in the conservative management of ankle arthritis. In cases of hypomobility of the ankle and surrounding soft tissues, orthoses are designed to transfer weight-bearing demands to adjacent flexible joints. With hypermobility leading to ankle joint degeneration from malalignment, the goal of orthoses is to realign the joints and limit this excessive motion.[13] Shoegear is commonly modified to include a rocker bottom sole in cases of ankle arthritis. This assists the patient with sagittal plane motion while limiting midfoot stress and increasing the propulsive forces of gait. Bracing is used when trying to substantially limit motion in the ankle in severe cases of arthritis where even minimal joint movement can elicit pain. The goal of the brace is to limit sagittal plane motion and stabilize the joint in a neutral position. A gauntlet ankle-foot orthosis (AFO) is the gold standard brace for this condition.[14] Some patients can function with a hinged AFO that can control the degree of motion at the ankle joint. This allows for some limit of motion without putting excess stress on other joints.[15] It is important to keep in mind that as the degree of ankle arthritis and associated deformity worsens, there is an increase in forces transmitted through the hindfoot. This can lead to early degenerative changes in both the subtalar and talonavicular joint, which is why bracing and shoe modifications can be of great importance in the treatment of ankle arthritis.

INJECTION THERAPY

Injection therapy for the conservative management of ankle joint osteoarthritis is a well-studied treatment modality with favorable outcomes.[16] There are several options for injectables in the treatment of ankle arthritis. Traditionally, injection therapy has been limited to the use of corticosteroid and anesthetic medications focused on the management of pain and inflammation. Recently with the advancements in biomedical technology and a focus toward regenerative medicine, biologic injection therapy has continued to grow in popularity. These additional injection therapies include the use of hyaluronic acid (HA), platelet-rich plasma (PRP), and various amniotic tissue derived (ATD) injections, which will serve as the focus of our discussion.

As with all injection therapies, the use of image guidance such as US may be of benefit to ensure the appropriate placement of the medication, particularly in end-stage arthritic joints with notable deformity. The following is the preferred technique for injection placement.[15]

- Iodine prep to the anterior medial shoulder: Measure site 1 cm from the tip of the medial malleolus and just medial to the tibialis anterior tendon
- With the ankle in dorsiflexion to protect the talar articular surface, the needle is directed approximately 45° lateral and into the anterior capsular pouch.

ANTI-INFLAMMATORIES

There are several kinds of anti-inflammatory medications that can be used to help treat the symptoms of ankle arthritis. Typical oral agents include non-steroidal anti-inflammatories (NSAIDs) and steroids. NSAIDs work by inhibiting cyclo-oxygenase (COX) enzymes, thus reducing the expression of proinflammatory cytokines. While these medications help to reduce inflammation and pain, they are associated with many negative side effects with chronic use.[17] The use of topical NSAIDs for treatment in ankle arthritis has shown to be efficacious with fewer adverse events due to lower systemic absorption.[18] Steroids work to control inflammation through immunosuppression, inhibiting the synthesis of inflammatory proteins by suppressing the genes that encode them. Oral steroids therefore work at a systemic level and while they may help with symptom relief, they are not without side effects.[19]

The use of injectable corticosteroids in the treatment of ankle arthritis is a well-studied practice which has been implemented for decades.[20] Corticosteroid injections specifically function to reduce intra-articular inflammation which results in a reduction in pain or symptoms. Dissimilar to biologic injections such as HA, PRP, or ATD, these injections lack any regenerative properties and only function to reduce symptoms and allow for more tolerable or pain-free motion. Several corticosteroids have been approved by the Food and Drug Administration (FDA) for intra-articular ankle injections, including methylprednisolone acetate (Depo-medrol), triamcinolone acetate (Kenalog 10, Kenalog 40), betamethasone acetate and betamethasone sodium phosphate (Celestone Soluspan), triamcinolone hexacetonide (Aristospan), and dexamethasone (dexamethasone sodium phosphate).[21] The use of these is well documented in the literature, with similar results for each individual steroid. Grice and colleagues reported that 86% of patients had significant improvement in symptoms with 29% remaining asymptomatic at 2 year follow up.[20] Ward and colleagues collected Foot and Ankle Outcome Scores before and after injection, and found significant improvement in scores post-injection. If patients still had pain relief at 2 months, it was predictive of sustained response at up to 1 year.[22]

There are few side effects associated with corticosteroid injections, including steroid flare, skin reaction, and infection, however, they are all relatively uncommon. Anderson and colleagues looked at 1708 patients who had intra-articular injections, and found only 5.8% to have adverse events.[23] Another possible negative effect is linked to acetate-based steroids, with the potential to catalyze further cartilage degeneration within the ankle.[24] Patient selection remains critical when determining the safety of repeated acetate based injections, and this treatment option may be suitable for only those with end-stage disease. Ankle arthritides which are mild to moderate and particularly inflammatory in nature traditionally demonstrate the greatest response to corticosteroid injection therapy, given the primary mechanism of action of the steroid in reducing inflammation.

HYALURONIC ACID

The early applications of viscosupplementation with HA as a nonoperative treatment option originally began with its use in the treatment of knee osteoarthritis.[25–28] Since that time, HA has also been utilized for the treatment of ankle osteoarthritis as well as many other synovial joints throughout the body.[29–32] At the current time, only the use of HA for the treatment of knee osteoarthritis is currently recognized by the FDA, though, off-label application in the ankle is now becoming more prevalent.

HA represents a vital component of the synovial fluid by contributing to the elasticity and viscosity of the fluid. It also serves as an extracellular matrix of articular cartilage and functions as a fluid shock absorber while also maintaining the structural and functional characteristics of the cartilage matrix.[33] On a cellular level, HA also serves many functions through the inhibition of prostaglandin formation and release, proteoglycan aggregation and synthesis, and modulation of the inflammatory response.[34] In the condition of osteoarthritis, the average molecular size and concentration of HA in the synovial fluid is diminished which ultimately leads to an increased vulnerability to cartilage damage. The utilization of intra-articular HA injections represents an effort to restore a more physiologically normal concentration of HA within the osteoarthritic joint. The function of HA serves primarily to reduce pain and inflammation while simultaneously supplementing the endogenous joint fluid. In addition, recent studies have also postulated that HA treatments may facilitate a biological activation due to the prolonged benefits of HA treatment following the initial injection.

Despite the plausible theories behind its usage, there is limited long-term literature supporting the application of HA in ankle osteoarthritis. Moreover, there remains a broad variability in the success of this modality based on the current reported literature.[35] Recent meta-analyses have demonstrated favorable outcomes in patients receiving intra-articular ankle HA injections.[35,36] Additional single-therapy studies have also reported beneficial outcomes with HA injections in patients with mild to moderate osteoarthritis.[29,30] In contrast to the aforementioned studies, a recent double-blind, randomized, and placebo controlled study demonstrated no clinical improvement when intra-articular HA injections were compared to a saline control group.[37] In addition to differing results in patient outcomes, there is significant variance in the dose and frequency of HA injections in the current literature.[38] Despite the lack of conclusive evidence reported on the efficacy of this treatment modality, no current literature reports adverse findings in regards to the safety of HA injections in ankle osteoarthritis. At this time we are unable to make specific treatment recommendations due to the paucity of substantial data and the current FDA consensus regarding the use of HA in the treatment of ankle osteoarthritis.

PLATELET-RICH PLASMA

Similar to HA, PRP injection therapy is gaining popularity in both the nonsurgical and surgical treatment of ankle arthritis and osteochondral defects. PRP is an autologous blood product that is created through centrifuge-mediated concentration of autologous blood which results in a product containing high concentrations of platelets and numerous growth factors. Contained within the alpha granules of the concentrated platelets are several various growth factors and cytokines which are vital in maintaining or restoring joint homeostasis and the initiation of healing cascades. The quality of the PRP product is determined by platelet concentration which correlates to the quantity of growth factors available in the product. Platelet concentration is primarily determined by the method of PRP preparation and can fluctuate based on the type of PRP preparation kit and centrifugation system utilized, as well as the number of centrifugation steps involved. As a result, several concentrations and preparation techniques have been reported in the literature, and currently no consensus statement has been made regarding the optimal concentration or preparation methods.

Promising results have been shown with the use of intra-articular PRP injections in both hip and knee mild to moderate primary OA. In addition, recent studies have shown improved patient-reported outcome measures and functional scores in patients receiving PRP for the treatment of ankle OCDs with and without surgical management.[39] While several studies exist evaluating PRP in the treatment of OCDs of the ankle; studies evaluating this modality in global OA of the ankle are scarce. In a case series of 20 subjects, Fukawa and colleagues demonstrated improvement in both pain and function in patients receiving three PRP injections at 2-week intervals with a mean follow-up of 24 weeks.[40] Additionally these authors reported no serious adverse events amongst their 20 subject cohort. In contrast, a more recent multicenter, block-randomized, double-blinded, placebo-controlled clinical trial of 100 subjects receiving 2 ultrasound-guided PRP injections demonstrated no improvement in symptoms or function in ankles with OA.[41] Though several studies support its use, the utilization of PRP remains controversial and we are unable to make specific treatment recommendations due to the current lack of substantial data regarding the use of PRP in the treatment of ankle osteoarthritis.

AMNIOTIC TISSUE-DERIVED PRODUCTS

The use of amniotic tissue derivatives has gained significant interest in the past decade for the treatment of various orthopedic conditions including osteoarthritis.[42–45] These amniotic-derived products include amniotic membrane and amniotic fluid products which serve as a potential treatment option through the augmentation of joint inflammation and healing. These products are derived from cells which are obtained from the fetal elements; amnion, chorion, amniotic fluid, and the umbilical cord. The amniotic tissue derivative products which are manufactured from these elements are intended to alter and improve the cytokine and cellular environment of the osteoarthritic joint. In the setting of osteoarthritis there is an increased intra-articular concentration of several synovial fluid cytokines and pathways including IL-1α, IL-1β, IL-18, TNF-α, and complement.[46,47] Ultimately these cytokines and prostaglandins lead to an increase in cartilage degeneration through the upregulation of matrix metalloproteinase production from the chondrocytes. It is believed that these amniotic tissue-derived products impart their effect via the interleukin 1 receptor antagonist (IL-1RA) and IL-10 which work to inhibit the progression and formation of inflammation. In addition, these amniotic tissue derivatives products promote the expression of tissue inhibitors of matrix metalloproteinases (TIMPs) which reduce the chondrocyte production of matrix metalloproteinases which cause cartilage degeneration.[48]

Current literature has demonstrated promising results with the use of amniotic tissue derivatives in the treatment of foot and ankle conditions such as plantar fasciitis, tendinopathies, and wounds though investigations into its application in ankle osteoarthritis leaves much to be desired.[42–45] Currently there is no literature evaluating the use of amniotic tissue derivatives in ankle osteoarthritis and only two studies have been performed in the human model to date. In an initial pilot study by Vines and colleagues, patients receiving a single injection of amniotic suspension allograft demonstrated a mean increase in patient-reported outcome measures at 1 year follow-up, though no further statistical analysis was performed due to the limited sample size.[49] A later randomized control trial was performed by Farr and colleagues consisting of 200 subjects with KL grade 2 to 3 OA who received either HA, ASA, or a saline control. At 6 month follow-up, patients receiving ASA demonstrated superior results in patient-reported outcome measures and pain subscores when compared to those receiving HA or saline control.[50] Despite promising initial research, we are unable to make specific treatment recommendations due to the current lack of substantial data regarding the use of ATDs in the treatment of ankle osteoarthritis.

SUMMARY

Ankle arthritis is a debilitating condition which can lead to pain, dysfunction, and an overall reduction in quality of life. Fortunately, due to the continued advancements in medicine and technology, there exists a multitude of non-surgical treatment options which may serve as viable options for long or short-term relief. Understanding the benefits and limitations of the conservative options discussed in this article will better equip one in reducing pain and mitigating functional losses in the arthritic ankle. Ultimately the authors recommend a fluid combination of mechanical offloading, oral anti-inflammatories, and analgesics, as well as local anti-inflammatory and regenerative injection therapies, each of which is customized to the specific patient's needs.

CLINICS CARE POINTS

- Ankle arthritis affects approximately 2% to 5% of the population with the majority being caused by traumatic injury.
- Not all patients are surgical candidates due to comorbidities or socioeconomic factors and must rely on conservative treatment management for symptom relief.
- Ankle injections are given through the anterior medial shoulder with the ankle in dorsiflexion and the needle directed 45° lateral and into the anterior capsular pouch for medication delivery.
- Corticosteroids, hyaluronic acid, platelet-rich plasma, and amniotic tissue-derived products have demonstrated relatively good clinical outcomes for pain relief in patients.

DISCLOSURE

No funding was received for this publication and there are no conflicts of interest.

REFERENCES

1. Hayes BJ, Gonzalez T, Smith JT, et al. Ankle Arthritis: You Can't Always Replace It. J Am Acad Orthop Surg 2016;24(2):29–38.
2. Ritterman SA, Fellars TA, Digiovanni CW. Current thoughts on ankle arthritis. R I Med J 2013;96(3):30–3.
3. Hendren L, Beeson P. A review of the differences between normal and osteoarthritis articular cartilage in human knee and ankle joints. Foot 2009;19(3):171–6.
4. Saltzman CL, Salamon ML, Blanchard GM, et al. Epidemiology of ankle arthritis: report of a consecutive series of 639 patients from a tertiary orthopaedic center. Iowa Orthop J 2005;25:44–6.
5. Shibuya N, McAlister JE, Prissel MA, et al. Consensus statement of the American College of foot and ankle Surgeons: diagnosis and treatment of ankle arthritis. JFAS 2020;59(5):1019–31.
6. Grunfeld R, Aydogan U, Juliano P. Ankle arthritis: review of diagnosis and operative management. Med Clin North Am 2014;98(2):267–89.
7. Barg A, Pagenstert GI, Hugle T, et al. Ankle osteoarthritis: etiology, diagnostics, and classification. Foot Ankle Clin 2013;18(3):411–26.
8. Wilkinson VH, Rowbotham EL, Grainger AJ. Imaging in foot and ankle arthritis. Semin Musculoskelet Radiol 2016;20(2):167–74.
9. Dohn UM, Ejbjerg BJ, Hasselquist M, et al. Rheumatoid arthritis bone erosion volumes on CT and MRI: reliability and correlations with erosion scores on CT, MRI and radiography. Ann Rheum Dis 2007;66(10):1388–92.
10. Giannini S, Buda R, Faldini C, et al. The treatment of severe posttraumatic arthritis of the ankle joint. J Bone Joint Surg Am 2007;89(Suppl 3):15–28.

11. Takakura Y, Aoki T, Sugimoto K. The treatment for osteoarthritis of the ankle joint. Jpn J Joint Dis 1986;5:347–52.

12. Ottawa P. Ottawa Panel evidence-based clinical practice guidelines for electro-therapy and thermotherapy interventions in the management of rheumatoid arthritis in adults. Phys Ther 2004;84(11):1016–43.

13. McGuire JB. Arthritis and related diseases of the foot and ankle: rehabilitation and biomechanical considerations. Clin Podiatr Med Surg 2003;20(3):469–85.

14. John S, Bongiovanni F. Brace management for ankle arthritis. Clin Podiatr Med Surg 2009;26(2):193–7.

15. Gentile MA. Nonsurgical treatment of ankle arthritis. Clin Podiatr Med Surg 2017; 34(4):415–23.

16. Vannabouathong C, Del Fabbro G, Sales B, et al. Intra-articular injections in the treatment of symptoms from ankle arthritis: a systematic review. Foot Ankle Int 2018;39:1141–50.

17. Roth SH, Anderson S. The NSAID dilemma: managing osteoarthritis in high-risk patients. Phys Sportsmed 2011;39(3):62–74.

18. Rannou F, Pelletier JP, Pelletier JM. Efficacy and safety of topical NSAIDs in the management of osteoarthritis: evidence from real-life setting trials and surveys. Semin Arthritis Rheum 2016;45(4):S18–21.

19. Barnes PJ. How corticosteroids control inflammation. Br J Pharmacol 2006; 148(3):245–54.

20. Grice J, Marsland D, Smith G, et al. Efficacy of foot and ankle corticosteroid injections. Foot Ankle Int 2017;38(1):8–13.

21. Pekarek B, Osher L, Buck S, et al. Intra-articular corticosteroid injections: a critical literature review with up-to-date findings. Foot 2011;21(2):66–70.

22. Ward ST, Williams PL, Purkayastha S. Intra-articular corticosteroid injections in the foot and ankle: a prospective 1-year follow-up investigation. JFAS 2008;47(2): 138–44.

23. Anderson SE, Lubberts B, Strong AD, et al. Adverse events and their risk factors following intra-articular corticosteroid injections of the ankle or subtalar joint. Foot Ankle Int 2019;40(6):622–8.

24. Robion FC, Doize B, Boure L, et al. Use of synovial fluid markers of cartilage synthesis and turnover to study effects of repeated intra-articular administration of methylprednisolone acetate on articular cartilage in vivo. J Orthop Res 2001; 19(2):250–8.

25. Lo GH, LaValley M, McAlindon T, et al. Intra-articular hyaluronic acid in treatment of knee osteoarthritis: a meta-analysis. JAMA 2003;290(23):3115–21.

26. Arrich J, Piribauer F, Mad P, et al. Intra-articular hyaluronic acid for the treatment of osteoarthritis of the knee: systematic review and meta-analysis. CMAJ (Can Med Assoc J) 2005;172(8):1039–43.

27. Bannuru RR, Natov NS, Dasi UR, et al. Therapeutic trajectory following intra-articular hyaluronic acid injection in knee osteoarthritis: a meta-analysis. Osteoarthritis Cartilage 2011;19(6):611–9.

28. Bannuru RR, Natov NS, Obadan IE, et al. Therapeutic trajectory of hyaluronic acid versus corticosteroids in the treatment of knee osteoarthritis: a systematic review and meta-analysis. Arthritis Rheum 2009;61(12):1704–11.

29. Salk RS, Chang TJ, D'Costa WF, et al. Sodium hyaluronate in the treatment of osteoarthritis of the ankle: a controlled, randomized, double-blind pilot study. J Bone Joint Surg Am 2006;88(2):295–302.

30. Sun SF, Chou YJ, Hsu CW, et al. Efficacy of intra-articular hyaluronic acid in patients with osteoarthritis of the ankle: a prospective study. Osteoarthritis Cartilage 2006;14(9):867–74.

31. Conrozier T, Bertin P, Mathieu P, et al. Intra-articular injections of hylan G-F 20 in patients with symptomatic hip osteoarthritis: an open label, multicentre, pilot study. Clin Exp Rheumatol 2003;21(5):605–10.

32. Labbe M, Ridgeland E, Savoie FH, et al. The short-term efficacy of hyaluronic acid injections for the treatment of degenerative arthrosis of the shoulder. Arthroscopy 2003;19:S13–8.

33. Frizziero L, Govoni E, Bachin P. Intraarticular hyaluronic acid in the treatment of osteoarthritis of the knee: clinical and morphological study. Clin Exp Rheumatol 1998;16(4):441–9.

34. Adams ME, Atkinson MH, Lussier AJ, et al. The role of viscosupplementation with hylan G-F 20 (Synvisc) in the treatment of osteoarthritis of the knee: a Canadian multicenter trial comparing hylan G-F 20 alone, hylan G-F 20 with non-steroidal antiinflammatory drugs (NSAIDs) and NSAIDs alone. Osteoarthritis Cartilage 1995;3(4):213–25.

35. Papalia R, Albo E, Russo F, et al. The use of hyaluronic acid in the treatment of ankle osteoarthritis: a review of the evidence. J Biol Regul Homeost Agents 2017;31(4 Suppl 2):91–102.

36. Chang KV, Hsiao MY, Chen WS, et al. Effectiveness of intra-articular hyaluronic acid for ankle osteoarthritis treatment: a systematic review and meta-analysis. Arch Phys Med Rehab 2013;94(5):951–60.

37. DeGroot H, Uzunishvili S, Weir R, et al. Intra-articular injection of hyaluronic acid is not superior to saline solution injection for ankle arthritis: a randomized, double-blind, placebo-controlled study. J Bone Joint Surg Am 2012;94(1):2–8.

38. Tikiz C, Unlu Z, Sener A, et al. Comparison of efficacy of lower and higher molecular weight viscosupplementation in the treatment of hip osteoarthritis. Clin Rheumatol 2005;24(3):244–50.

39. Mei-Dan O, Carmont MR, Laver L, et al. Platelet-rich plasma or hyaluronate in the management of osteochondral lesions of the talus. Am J Sports Med 2012;40(3):534–41.

40. Fukawa T, Yamaguchi S, Akatsu Y, et al. Safety and efficacy of intra-articular injection of platelet-rich plasma in patients with ankle osteoarthritis. Foot Ankle Int 2017;38(6):596–604.

41. Paget LDA, Reurink G, de Vos R, et al. Effect of platelet-rich plasma injections vs placebo on ankle symptoms and function in patients with ankle osteoarthritis: a randomized clinical trial. JAMA 2021;326(16):1595–605.

42. Shah AP. Using amniotic membrane allografts in the treatment of neuropathic foot ulcers. J Am Podiatr Med Assoc 2014;104(2):198–202.

43. Swan J. Use of cryopreserved, particulate human amniotic membrane and umbilical cord (AM/UC) tissue: a case series study for application in the healing of chronic wounds. Surg Technol Int 2014;25:73–8.

44. DiDomenico LA, Orgill DP, Galiano RD, et al. Use of an aseptically processed, dehydrated human amnion and chorion membrane improves likelihood and rate of healing in chronic diabetic foot ulcers: a prospective, randomized, multi-centre clinical trial in 80 patients. Int Wound J 2018;15(6):950–7.

45. Sultan AA, Piuzzi NS, Mont MA. Nonoperative applications of placental tissue matrix in orthopaedic sports injuries. Clin J Sport Med 2020;30(4):383–9.

46. Kueckelhaus M, Philip J, Kamel RA, et al. Sustained release of amnion-derived cellular cytokine solution facilitates Achilles tendon healing in rats. Eplasty 2014;14:e29.

47. Lange-Consiglio A, Rossi D, Tassan S, et al. Conditioned medium from horse amniotic membrane-derived multipotent progenitor cells: immunomodulatory activity in vitro and first clinical application in tendon and ligament injuries in vivo. Stem Cells Dev 2013;22(22):3015–24.

48. Bennett NT, Schultz GS. Growth factors and wound healing: biochemical properties of growth factors and their receptors. Am J Surg 1993;165(6):728–37.

49. Vines J, Aliprantis AO, Gomoll AH, et al. Cryopreserved amniotic suspension for the treatment of knee osteoarthritis. J Knee Surg 2016;29(6):443–50.

50. Farr J, Gomoll AH, Yanke AB, et al. A randomized controlled single-blind study demonstrating superiority of amniotic suspension allograft injection over hyaluronic acid and saline control for modification of knee osteoarthritis symptoms. J Knee Surgery 2019;32(11):1143–54.

The Ankle Joint

Updates on Ankle Fusion Approaches and Fixation

Jason George DeVries, DPM*, Brandon M. Scharer, DPM

KEYWORDS

- Anterior approach • Transfibular • External fixation • Arthroscopic • Tibiotalar joint
- Replacement

KEY POINTS

- Ankle fusion is a reliable, predictable, and time-tested approach for ankle arthritis.
- Many options and approaches are available for ankle fusion, each with their own pros and cons.
- Comparison with ankle replacement is valid and both options should be discussed with patients.
- The recovery can be accelerated compared with historical timeframe because of approaches that are more protective of the local biology and blood supply, and improved fixation.

INTRODUCTION

Ankle arthrodesis is a well-studied, classical procedure for conditions affecting the ankle joint. It has been considered the gold standard for treatment of ankle arthritis, regardless of the cause of the joint damage.[1–4] The main indications for an ankle fusion include arthritis from any source, including septic arthritis, deformity, instability, trauma, and Charcot neuroarthropathy.[5] The utility of the procedure is demonstrated by the long history after being introduced in 1927[1] with at least 40 different operative techniques developed and its wide array of indications.[6] It is also indicated in patients with a wide variety of demographic, social, and past medical histories, although certain conditions are perceived to increase the risks in ankle arthrodesis, as is consistent with other surgical procedures.[7,8]

Although historical data have indicated up to a 40% nonunion rate,[9] more modern literature shows nonunion rate to be closer to 10%.[10] This is met out across open and arthroscopic approaches and a variety of fixation methods. In terms of an update on modern literature, there are two areas that have garnered particular attention. First is

Orthopedics and Sports Medicin - BayCare Clinic, 1110 Kepler Drive, Green Bay, WI 54311, USA
* Corresponding author.
E-mail address: jdevries@baycare.net

Clin Podiatr Med Surg 40 (2023) 681–701
https://doi.org/10.1016/j.cpm.2023.05.010
0891-8422/23/© 2023 Elsevier Inc. All rights reserved.

podiatric.theclinics.com

the use of anterior plating. This has been shown to have biomechanical advantages compared with crossed screw fixation,[11] and a systematic review of studies using anterior plating reported a 97.6% rate of union in 164 patients.[12] Several studies have also directly compared ankle fusion with anterior plating or crossed screws. Excellent fusion rates are noted with anterior plating having superior fusion rates, but without statistically significant differences in the groups.[13,14] The second area of focus is on open and arthroscopic approaches for ankle fusion. Arthroscopic ankle arthrodesis was first introduced in 1983[15] and has been shown to be effective in subsequent reports.[16,17] More recent analyses have systematically compared the open and arthroscopic approaches, and have found that fusion rate, blood loss, and tourniquet time are all improved in the arthroscopic approach.[18,19] In addition, the arthroscopic approach has been reported to have superior outcomes to an open approach in terms of functional outcomes and quality of life,[20] cost,[21] and need for subsequent adjacent joint procedures.[22] Recently new hardware options have been introduced that combine these two areas to allow for a minimal or arthroscopic approach with additional anterior plating.

In addition to evaluating specific approaches for ankle fusion, no discussion would be complete without a discussion of ankle fusion compared with ankle replacement. Although ankle fusion is often considered the gold standard, there are clear shifts toward ankle replacement. Trends have been evaluated and practice patterns have been reported previously. From 2004 to 2009 there was a 57% increase in performance of ankle replacement.[23] From 2007 to 2013 the share of patients having total ankle replacement for end-stage ankle arthritis was 14% in 2007 and increased to 45% by 2013. In particular, there was a 12-fold increase in the use of ankle replacement for posttraumatic ankle arthritis.[24] In a study published in 2022 looking at ankle fusion and replacement in New York and California from 2015 to 2018 the authors found that an equal number of replacements and fusions were performed.[25] Although there are advocates for ankle replacement in ever increasing parameters, a 2020 systematic review and meta-analysis shows no clear superior option when comparing replacement and fusion. The study looked at American Orthopaedic Foot and Ankle Society (AOFAS), visual analog scale, and ankle osteoarthritis scale scores, and several other parameters. There was no significant difference in AOFAS total, pain and alignment scores, visual analog scale and ankle osteoarthritis scale scores, gait analysis, and satisfaction rate between groups. The replacement group had better AOFAS function scores and range of motion outcomes. However, the ankle fusion group had fewer complications and a lower reoperation rate.[26] Although ankle replacement is becoming more common, there is clearly still a place for ankle fusion.

Although there are many different historical approaches and methods of fixation for ankle fusion, there are now a few different approaches that make up most procedures and represent the current state of the art. This article is an update to present current approaches for ankle fusion performed arthroscopically, open with crossed screws, open with an anterior plate, and with external fixation.

ARTHROSCOPIC ANKLE ARTHRODESIS
Indications

Arthroscopic ankle arthrodesis is more preserving to the local vascularity, more anatomically sparing, and has excellent union rates and satisfaction. It is indicated and the preferred approach in patients with arthritis of the ankle joint with limited coronal plane deformity, a mobile joint, and osteophyte formation small enough to allow for introduction of arthroscopic equipment. It is beneficial in patients with a poor soft tissue envelope (including skin grafts or flaps) that would be at risk in open procedures. This approach can also be considered in patients in whom cosmetic appearance is important. It is often used in patients that would otherwise be candidates for ankle replacement that have contraindications, such as a young age or weight. There are also relative contraindications. Because of the limited approach and bone-sparing nature it may be more difficult to correct angular deformity and is more difficult to deal with large bony defects. Ankles with very large anterior spurring, or severe arthrofibrosis may also make entry into the ankle and maneuvering of the instrumentation more difficult. Experience and comfort level with the procedure can overcome these difficulties and has been reported in large coronal plane deformity,[27] stiff joints,[28] loss of the lateral malleolus,[29] and others.

Case Study and Technique

A 38-year-old man presented with left ankle pain. He had three previous ankle surgeries in the last 3 years: two ankle arthroscopies and an arthrotomy for osteochondral defect with Dwyer osteotomy. The most recent arthroscopy was 5 months before presentation and he was told that the joint was grossly arthritic. The patient had less than 15° of total ankle range of motion and was a hunting and fishing guide. Surrounding joints at the talonavicular and subtalar were in good condition (**Fig. 1**). An arthroscopic ankle arthrodesis was chosen.

The patient is placed on the operating table in the supine position. A thigh holder and noninvasive distraction is applied. This allows for easier access to the posterior aspect of the joint. Standard anterior-medial and anterior-lateral portals are made, and the arthroscope is introduced. Once the joint is identified, a posterior-lateral portal is made at the level of the joint from adjacent to the Achilles. Through this portal a

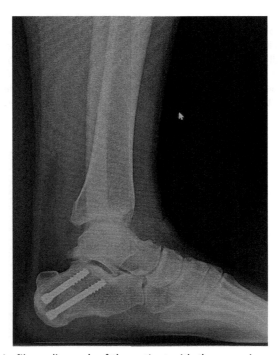

Fig. 1. Lateral plain film radiograph of the patient with three previous ankle surgeries.

dedicated inflow cannula is introduced. This is used to allow for unimpeded inflow, and to flush any joint debris from the posterior recess of the joint (**Fig. 2**).

Joint debridement is started with a 4.0-mm shaver to remove fibrosis, synovitis, and cartilage (**Fig. 3**). This softer material is not efficiently removed with a burr. Any impinging osteophytes should be identified and removed at this time. A burr or even osteotome may be used. This opens the working space to remove the cartilage. Work systematically to remove the cartilage from the anterior talus, medial and lateral gutters, and tibia. The posterior aspect of the talus is typically not accessible with a straight or even curved shaver. Angled curettes are used to remove the cartilage from the posterior talus (**Fig. 4**), with frequent use of the shaver to removal cartilaginous debris. The curettes can also be used to free up the soft tissues along the posterior ankle joint as necessary. At this point the joint should be open with diastasis across the joint and easy accessibility throughout.

A 4.0 to 5.0 barrel-shaped burr is then used to remove the subchondral bone plate. Again, it is imperative to work systematically (**Fig. 5**). Penetration past the subchondral plate should be performed throughout the joint. However, care must be taken to preserve the overall shape of the joint to allow good bony apposition and ensure that the joints will compress with fixation. Overly aggressive preparation does not allow for bony contact with compression. If any coronal plant deformity needs to be corrected, it is done with the burr. Once the joint is prepared past the subchondral bone, the burr is penetrated more deeply in several areas to fenestrate the joint surface. Arthroscopic awls and guidewires are used to fenestrate the area throughout.

After the joint is prepared, fixation is started. Typically, three screws at 6.5 mm or larger are used. With the arthroscope still in the joint and distraction applied, guidewires are introduced (**Fig. 6**). Two medial wires are placed from proximal to the medial malleolus angled into the joint. The goal is to maximize the anterior to posterior spread to allow for a broad footprint of fixation. The pins are visualized in the joint with the arthroscope to confirm good placement. The pins are then pulled back under the tibial joint space. A third wire is then introduced from the lateral tibia. This should be placed anterior to the fibula and centrally between the medial wires. Again, visualization confirms good placement of the wire, and the wire is pulled back. Confirmation with fluoroscopy is performed. After the wires are placed, orthobiologics, such as demineralized bone matrix, is placed through the posterior inflow cannula and visualized (**Fig. 7**).

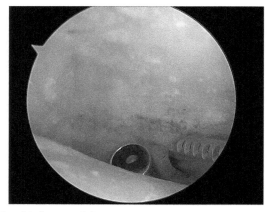

Fig. 2. Posterior-lateral inflow portal.

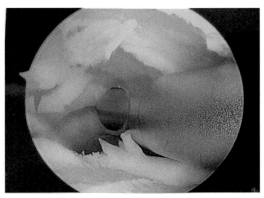

Fig. 3. Arthroscopic shaver for initial removal of fibrosis and articular cartilage.

The noninvasive distraction is released, and the leg is taken out of the thigh holder. The foot and ankle are held in position and compressed, and the guidewires are advanced into the talus. Appropriate position is confirmed clinically and fluoroscopically. Screws are then applied and compressed (**Fig. 8**). There may still be gap apparent on the images, which is common.

Technical Pearls

- Posterior-lateral inflow portal to flush posterior joint and allow for high volume inflow.
- Angled curettes are used to access and prepare the posterior talus.
- Visualize the guidewires in the joint to confirm good placement and spread, then pull them back to allow positioning.
- Apply orthobiologics through the posterior cannula before release of distraction.

OPEN TRANSFIBULAR ANKLE ARTHRODESIS
Indications

The traditional approach for ankle fusion is from a combined lateral and medial approach. The fibula is osteotomized and reflected posteriorly for lateral onlay graft

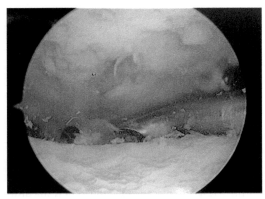

Fig. 4. Angled curettes are used to remove the articular surface from the posterior aspect of the talus.

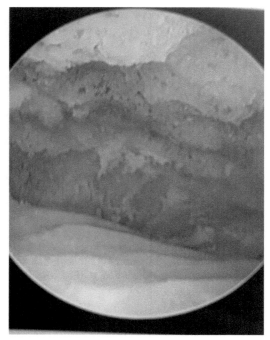

Fig. 5. A systematic approach is used to remove any remaining articular surface past the subchondral bone with a burr.

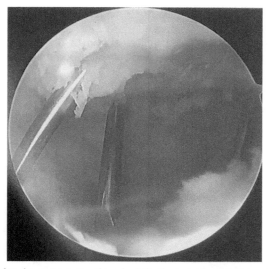

Fig. 6. Guidewires for the screws are placed while the joint is still distracted to visualize the placement and spread of the screws. These are then pulled back into the tibia for positioning after distraction is released.

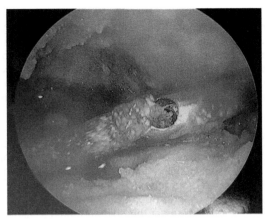

Fig. 7. Orthobiologics are introduced through the posterior inflow portal before release of the noninvasive distraction.

with the medial half morselized for use as autogenous graft. It is usually fixated with crossed screws, but a lateral plate can be used. It is indicated in patients that have large deformity in the coronal or sagittal plane. It can also correct translational issue, such as significant anterior or posterior displacement of the talus on the tibia. Patients that require work at the fibula for such issues as hardware, infection, or deformity correction should be addressed with the transfibular approach to avoid multiple

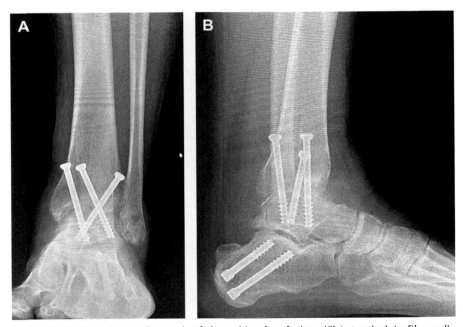

Fig. 8. (*A*) Mortise plain radiograph of the ankle after fusion. (*B*) Lateral plain film radiograph of the ankle after fusion.

incisions near each other. Because of the likely injury to the peroneal artery, it is contraindicated in patients with tenuous blood supply. Expect swelling and stiffness after this approach as well from vascular insult and multiple incisions. Patients need to have reasonable expectation on cosmesis with large incisions and change in bony structure from the fibular osteotomy. Finally, caution should be used with how much fibula is left, in what condition, and in what position if there is any potential for takedown to total ankle replacement. Loss of the fibula is a strong contraindication for later ankle replacement.[30]

Case Study and Technique

A 54-year-old, 300-lb truck driver presented to the clinic with ankle pain. This was found to be not only arthritic, but also had significant anterior extrusion (**Fig. 9**). After failing conservative measures, surgery was offered. The patient was scheduled for ankle fusion because of his weight, age, and activity level. A transfibular approach was chosen to allow for planar cuts at the tibia and talus to allow for posterior positioning of the talus under the tibia. In this case, a plate was chosen as well.

Patient is placed on the table in the supine position. The foot is placed into a slightly adducted position to the standard toes up position. This allows easier access to the lateral ankle where most of the work is done. A 12-cm incision is made laterally over the fibula. Dissection is carried down and the fibula is identified. The anterior attachments and anterior-inferior tibiofibular ligament are transected. The fibula is then osteotomized in an oblique fashion 5-cm proximal to the joint (**Fig. 10**). A second osteotomy is made, and a 1-cm section of fibula is removed. This is to prevent impingement laterally. The fibula is then distracted away from the tibia with a laminar

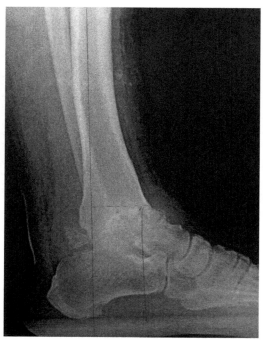

Fig. 9. Lateral plain radiograph of the patient with significant anterior extrusion of the talus from the tibia.

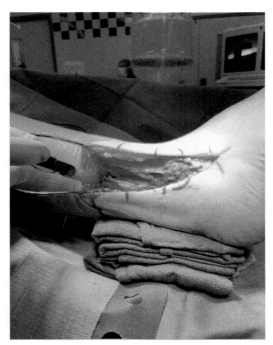

Fig. 10. Sagittal saw is used to perform an oblique osteotomy above the level of the ankle joint. A second osteotomy is then used to remove approximately 1 cm of fibula to allow for shortening.

spreader or Gelpi retractor. The medial half of the fibula is then removed with a sagittal saw and morselized for bone graft (**Fig. 11**). A second incision is then made anterior-medially along the gutter of the ankle joint. This allows access to the medial ankle.

Once exposure is made, the joint is prepared in either curettage or planar cuts technique. Because this approach is more often made for revision or severely deformed cases, planar cuts are more common. A sagittal saw is used to remove the articular surface of the tibia for deformity correction. This is done with fluoroscopic and visual confirmation medially to protect the medial malleolus. Through the medial incision, the articular portion of the medial malleolus is removed with a saw. The foot is then positioned into proper alignment, and a saw is used to prepare the dorsal and medial aspect of the talus to allow for deformity correction and good bony apposition (**Fig. 12**). The lateral articular surface of the talus is then removed.

The joint is then packed and positioned. Typically, slight posterior position allows for a shorter anterior lever arm and a more natural gait. Planar cuts make this easy. In this case, the talus was significantly posteriorly translated to position the lateral talar process under the axis of the tibia. Once positioned, the area is pinned into place. Screw placement is similar to the arthroscopic approach, and then the fibula is placed back into place with a screw above and below the joint. If a lateral plate is used as in this case, fibula onlay may not be possible (**Fig. 13**).

Technical Pearls

- Remove a 1-cm section of fibula at the osteotomy to allow for shortening and prevent lateral impingement.

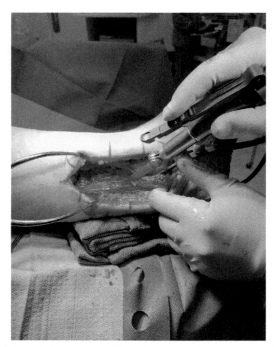

Fig. 11. The medial side of the retracted fibula is removed with a saw and morselized to use as bone graft and to create a raw surface for fusion.

- Planar cuts allow for deformity correction, including posterior positioning of the talus.
- Screw fixation of the ankle is standard, with fibula onlay grafting fixated with a screw above and below the ankle joint.

OPEN ANTERIOR ANKLE ARTHRODESIS WITH PLATE
Indications

Anterior ankle arthrodesis is the preferred approach for patients with frontal plane deformity and sufficient soft tissue envelop. This is an excellent approach for patients with contraindications to total ankle replacement, including peripheral neuropathy, incompetent deltoid ligament/stage IV posterior tibial tendon dysfunction, and talar avascular necrosis. The approach and technique have improved over recent years with precontoured plating and fixation systems similar to the first metatarsal phalangeal joint. The most important benefit to this approach is maintaining the fibula and fibular length in younger patients, which allows for possible take down total ankle replacement (TAR) in the future if needed. The anterior surgical approach for ankle fusion makes any future TAR procedures optimal for placement.

Case Study and Technique

A 51-year-old man complained of ankle pain after previous ankle fracture and fixation. After failing conservative measures, the patient was evaluated for either ankle fusion or replacement (**Fig. 14**). Preoperative computed tomography (CT) scan revealed significant posttraumatic arthritis, but also a large lateral talar cyst (**Fig. 15**). The patient was

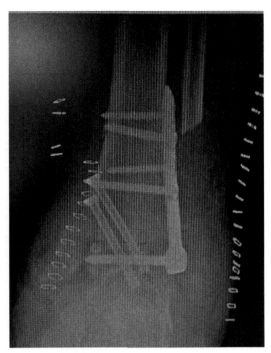

Fig. 12. Immediate postoperative radiograph shows the intersecting planar cuts used to create a broad flat surface. This allows for deformity correction bony contact.

deemed to not have adequate talar bone stock for a TAR, and anterior ankle fusion with plate was chosen. This allowed for direct access to the cyst for grafting.

The patient is brought to the operating room and placed on the operating table in the supine position. Attention is directed to the anterior aspect of the ankle. Here a 15-cm incision was made directly anteriorly along the midline of the ankle. This is done in a longitudinal fashion. An interval should be attempted to be made just medial to the extensor hallucis longus tendon. Dissection should be carried deep through subcutaneous tissue. Next, through meticulous dissection the incision is carried down to the level of the ankle joint capsule. The capsule is opened in a linear fashion and all capsular and periosteal tissues are dissected free of their osseous attachments and reflected medially and laterally, exposing the ankle joint to the operative field. Any spurs should be removed with a combination rongeur and osteotomes. The joint is then distracted and prepared for fusion. This is done with the combination of rongeur, osteotomes, and 4.0-mm ball burr. All remaining articular cartilage is removed down past the subchondral bone. Any deformity should be corrected through bone removal at this level. Sagittal saw is used sparingly only if the deformity cannot be corrected through curettage. Sagittal saw should be used to remove a portion of the fibula to decompress the joint. In this patient, the talar dome was also opened with a quarter-inch osteotome laterally to allow access to the large talar cyst. The cyst was curettaged and was grafted with allogeneic bone morphogenetic protein-2 with cancellous chips.

The medial and lateral gutters of the ankle joint should also be prepared for arthrodesis. After removal of the articular surface passed the subchondral bone, the area should further be prepared for fusion by fenestration with a solid drill (**Fig. 16**). Finally,

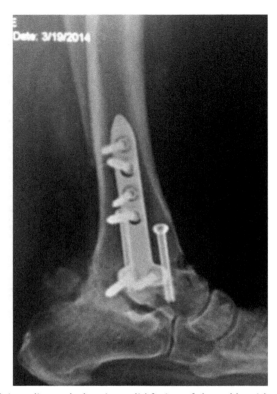

Fig. 13. Lateral plain radiograph showing solid fusion of the ankle with a lateral plate. The talus has been moved posteriorly to be under the tibia.

the subchondral plate should be scaled using quarter-inch osteotome. All this is done to facilitate a raw, bleeding bone surface. The bone fragments are left in place. The area is compressed and a guidewire from a large, cannulated screw is placed from proximal to the medial malleolus into the talus and a compression screw is applied across the fusion site. The anterior compression plate is applied with distal screws in the talus applied first, followed by the dynamic compression slot in the tibia. The precontoured plate guides the ankle position, but sometimes the tibia or talus needs to be contoured to allow the plate to sit flush (**Fig. 17**). Postoperative radiographs and CT scans showed solid fusion of the ankle and good fill of the talar cyst (**Figs. 18** and **19**).

Technical Pearls

- Deep dissection should be made just medial to the extensor hallucis longus to avoid the neurovascular bundle.
- Coronal plane correction is easily observed from the anterior approach and should be corrected with curettage technique, avoiding sagittal saw use if possible, to maintain the curvature of the joint.
- Initial medial compression screw placement obtains initial position and compression, which is then aided and slightly changed with anterior plate.
- Maintaining anatomy and landmarks at the medial and lateral gutters allows for technical assistance in the need for future TAR.

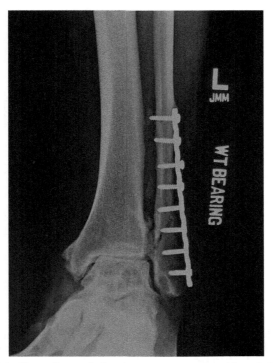

Fig. 14. Mortise plain film radiograph showing posttraumatic ankle arthritis, mild varus, and lucency in the talar body.

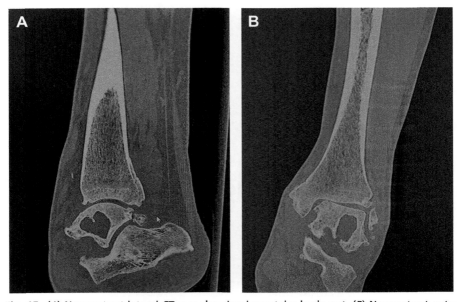

Fig. 15. (*A*) Noncontrast lateral CT scan showing large talar body cyst. (*B*) Noncontrast anteroposterior CT scan showing incongruent varus ankle arthritis and large lateral talar body cyst.

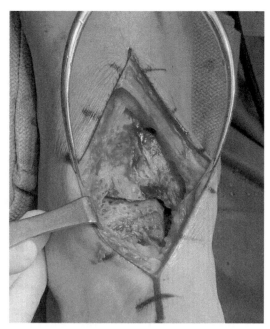

Fig. 16. Anterior incision with interval between the tibialis anterior and extensor hallucis longus. Anterior tibial bone spurs have been removed, articular surface has been prepared, and the fusion site is fenestrated.

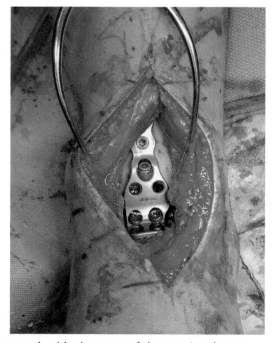

Fig. 17. Anterior approach with placement of the anterior plate.

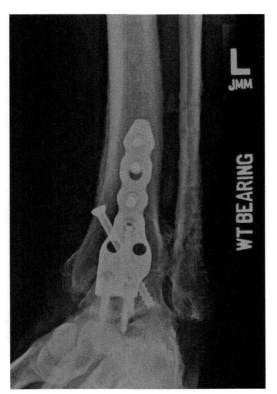

Fig. 18. Mortise plain film radiograph showing varus correction, maintenance of the medial and lateral gutters, and solid ankle joint fusion.

EXTERNAL FIXATION ANKLE ARTHRODESIS
Indications

Regardless of surgical approach and arthrodesis technique, there are circumstances where traditional internal fixation is not possible. External fixation with compression has been used in many forms for ankle fusion. Specific configurations can allow for gradual correction, postoperative adjustments, and may be placed in single and multiple planes. Indications for external fixation are typically in cases where internal fixation is not possible. Poor soft tissue coverage from previous or current trauma may necessitate external fixation. Infection and osteomyelitis are also contraindications for internal fixation and may require external hardware. If there is deformity that cannot be corrected at the index procedure and requires gradual correction over time, internal hardware is not possible. Significant bone loss, such as collapse of the talus in avascular necrosis, may not have enough bone fixate internally, and external fixation can address this. There are significant downsides to using external fixation, and this must be weighed when considering this method. Pin tract infection is common.[31] It is most often easily treated with local wound care and oral antibiotics, but can progress and require early removal or develop into a bony infection. Large pins in the bones, especially in the tibia, can lead to stress risers and even overt fractures.[32] Patients may have a difficult time tolerating the device, which can lead to early removal.

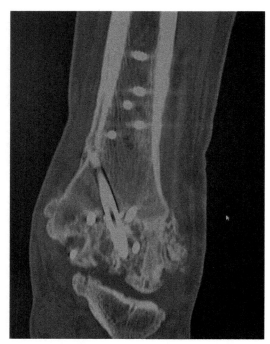

Fig. 19. Coronal plane noncontrast CT confirming solid fusion at the ankle joint and bony fill of the lateral talar cyst.

Case Study and Technique

A 28-year-old man had a history of an ankle arthroscopy 7 months before presentation. The surgery was complicated by infection and draining sinus. Before presentation the ankle was managed with an arthroscopic washout and debridement, and later a bone biopsy. The biopsy was positive for osteomyelitis of the tibia, talus, and fibula. MRI was also read as osteomyelitis and severe articular cartilage loss and arthritis **(Fig. 20)**. However, his laboratory values were essentially normal without elevation of white blood cell count, erythrocyte sedimentation rate, or C-reactive protein. Therefore, a white blood cell–labeled bone scan was ordered, which showed uptake at the ankle without white blood cell collection at the ankle. In consultation with infectious disease, a larger biopsy with culture was recommended and performed. This resulted in *Propionibacterium acnes* being cultured in the fibula and talus. Infectious disease recommended against any internal hardware, and the patient was scheduled for septic ankle fusion with circular external fixation.

Any joint preparation is acceptable, and this patient had an arthroscopic joint preparation. Once prepared, the joint was pinned into place and the fixation was applied. This was meant as definitive fixation and circular fixator was chosen. A foot plate was placed with wires in the calcaneus, metatarsals, and a post from the plate for wires into the talus. Two circular rings were placed into the tibia with crossed wire technique only to try to minimize potential for tibial stress fracture with half pins. Compression was then applied from the distal tibial plate to the foot plate **(Fig. 21)**.

Patient was allowed to start protected weight bearing at the 2-week postoperative visit. Patient was placed on continued suppressive antibiotics by infectious disease. At

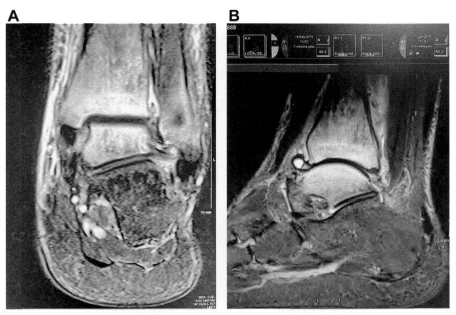

Fig. 20. (*A*) Coronal plane T2-weighted MRI showing uptake in the talus, tibia, and fibula. This was read as osteomyelitis. (*B*) Sagittal T2-weighted MRI showing uptake in the tibia and talus with anterior effusion.

approximately 10 weeks the external fixator was removed, and the patient was placed into a boot for 1 month. Patient had delayed union and was left on suppressive antibiotics. A bone stimulator was prescribed and 10 months after the ankle fusion a CT scan confirmed a solid but approximately 50% partial union of the ankle (**Fig. 22**).

Technical Pearls

- External fixation is used in extenuating circumstances where internal fixation is not viable.
- Any method of joint preparation is acceptable as long as the joint can be prepared and positioned before external fixation.

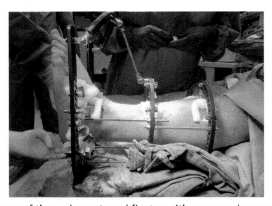

Fig. 21. Clinical image of three-ring external fixator with compression across the ankle joint.

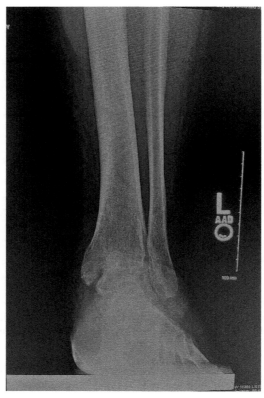

Fig. 22. Anteroposterior plain radiograph showing fusion of the ankle joint after removal of the external fixator.

- A post from the foot plate into the talus allows for compression across the ankle without compression at the subtalar joint.
- External fixation allows for postoperative adjustments, such as compression.

RECOVERY

At 2 weeks postoperatively, the Plaster of Paris splint and the dressings are removed. Radiographs are taken, the wound is checked, sutures are removed, and the area is redressed, and a fiberglass cast is then applied. At 6 weeks postoperatively, patients are seen again for a radiograph. At this time, patients are placed in a pneumatic boot, continue non-weight-bearing, and begin range of motion exercises. Patients then return at 8 weeks for radiographs and begin full weight-bearing in the boot. Patients then return at 12 weeks for radiographs and return to normal shoe gear. Following this visit, the patient returns in 8 weeks for final radiographs. If they are symptomatic with continued pain, then a weight-bearing CT scan is obtained.

COMPLICATIONS

As with any joint arthrodesis, nonunion is the most common complication and no different with the ankle joint. The modern literature nonunion rate is around 10%.[10]

If union is achieved, malalignment and malunion is another unfortunate complication and difficult for the patient. The most significant malalignment observed is internal rotation and varus, and the second most severe is equinus. This can produce significant gait problems and must be avoided. This is aided with the advent of precontoured anterior plate designs, which help reduce this risk and other complications.

SUMMARY

Ankle arthrodesis is a well-studied, classical procedure for conditions affecting the ankle joint. It has been considered the historical gold standard for treatment of ankle arthritis, regardless of the cause of the joint damage.[1-4] Although total ankle replacement is now the new gold standard for treating end-stage ankle arthritis, ankle arthrodesis still has its indications. Although there are many different historical approaches and methods of fixation for ankle fusion, certain approaches are preferred based on patient needs. New techniques and approaches allow for improved efficiencies and abilities to maintain the fibula for future surgical indications if needed.

CLINICS CARE POINTS

Arthroscopic Ankle Fusion
- Posterior-lateral inflow portal to flush posterior joint and allow for high-volume inflow.
- Angled curettes are used to access and prepare the posterior talus.
- Visualize the guidewires in the joint to confirm good placement and spread, then pull them back to allow positioning.
- Apply orthobiologics through the posterior cannula before release of distraction.

Transfibular Open Ankle Fusion
- Remove a 1-cm section of fibula at the osteotomy to allow for shortening and prevent lateral impingement.
- Planar cuts allow for deformity correction, including posterior positioning of the talus.
- Screw fixation of the ankle is standard, with fibula onlay grafting fixated with a screw above and below the ankle joint.

Anterior Ankle Arthrodesis
- Deep dissection should be made just medial to the extensor hallucis longus to avoid the neurovascular bundle.
- Coronal plane correction is easily observed from the anterior approach and should be corrected with curettage technique, avoiding sagittal saw use if possible, to maintain the curvature of the joint.
- Initial medial compression screw placement obtains initial position and compression, which is then aided and slightly changed with anterior plate.
- Maintaining anatomy and landmarks at the medial and lateral gutters allows for technical assistance in the need for future TAR.

DISCLOSURE

Dr J.G. DeVries is design consultant for Nextremity.

REFERENCES

1. Straub G. Arthrodesis of the ankle. Surg Gynecol Obstet 1927;45:676.
2. Smith R, Wood P. Arthrodesis of the ankle in the presence of a large deformity in the coronal plane. JBJS Br 2007;89-B:615–9.

3. Ferkel RD, Hewitt M. Long-term results of arthroscopic ankle arthrodesis. Foot Ankle Int 2005;26:275–80.

4. Holt ES, Hansen ST, Mayo KA, et al. Ankle arthrodesis using internal screw fixation. Clin Orthop Relat Res 1991;268:21–8.

5. Dujela MD, Hyer CF. Ankle arthrodesis: open anterior and arthroscopic approaches. In: Hyer CF, Berlet GC, Philbin TM, et al, editors. Essential foot and ankle surgical techniques: a multidisciplanry approach. 1st edition. Switzerland: Springer Nature; 2019. p. 275–90.

6. Helm R. The results of ankle arthrodesis. J Bone Joint Surg Br 1990;72:141–3.

7. Thevendran G, Shah K, Pinney SJ, et al. Perceived risk factors for nonunion following foot and ankle arthrodesis. J Orthop Surg 2017;25:1–6.

8. Chalayon O, Wang B, Blankenhorn B, et al. Factors affecting the outcomes of uncomplicated primary open ankle arthrodesis. Foot Ankle Int 2015;36:1170–9.

9. Frey C, Halikus NM, Vu-Rose T, et al. A review of ankle arthrodesis: predisposing factors to nonunion. Foot Ankle Int 1994;15(11):581–4.

10. Yasui Y, Hannon CP, Seow D, et al. Ankle arthrodesis: a systematic approach and review of the literature. World J Orthop 2016;7(11):700–8.

11. Betz MM, Benninger EE, Favre PP, et al. Primary stability and stiffness in ankle arthrodes: crossed screws versus anterior plating. Foot Ankle Surg 2013; 19(30):168–72.

12. Kusnezov N, Dunn JC, Koehler LR, et al. Anatomically contoured anterior plating for isolated tibiotalar arthrodesis: a systematic review. Foot Ankle Spec 2017;10: 352–8.

13. Mitchell PM, Douleh DG, Thomson AB. Comparison of ankle fusion rates with and without anterior plate augmentation. Foot Ankle Int 2017;38:419–23.

14. Prissel MA, Simpson GA, Sutphen SA, et al. Ankle arthrodesis: a retrospective analysis comparing single column, locked anterior plating to crossed lag screw technique. J Foot Ankle Surg 2017;56:453–6.

15. Schneider D. Arthroscopic ankle fusion. Arthroscopic Video J 1983;3.

16. Gougoulias NE, Agathangelidis FG, Parsons SW. Arthroscopic ankle arthrodesis. Foot Ankle Int 2007;28(6):695–706.

17. Collman DR, Kaas MH, Schuberth JM. Arthroscopic ankle arthrodesis: factors influencing union in 39 consecutive patients. Foot Ankle Int 2006;27(12):1079–85.

18. Bai Z, Yang Y, Chen S, et al. Clinical effectiveness of arthroscopic vs open ankle arthrodesis for advanced ankle arthritis: a systematic review and meta-analysis. Medicine 2021;100:10.

19. Mok TN, He Q, Panneerselavam S, et al. Open versus arthroscopic ankle arthrodesis: a systematic review and meta-analysis. J Orthop Surg Res 2020;15:187–99.

20. Berk TA, van Baal MCPM, Sturkenboom JM, et al. Functional outcomes and quality of life in patients with post-traumatic arthrosis undergoing open or arthroscopic talocrural arthrodesis: a retrospective cohort with prospective follow-up. J Foot Ankle Surg 2022;61:609–14.

21. Peterson KS, Lee MS, Buddecke DE. Arthroscopic versus open ankle arthrodesis: a retrospective cost analysis. J Foot Ankle Surg 2010;49:242–7.

22. Yasui Y, Vig KS, Murawski CD, et al. Open versus arthroscopic ankle arthrodesis: a comparison of subsequent procedures in a large database. J Foot Ankle Surg 2016;55:777–81.

23. Terrell RD, Montgomery SR, Pannell WC, et al. Comparison of practice patterns in total ankle replacement and ankle fusion in the United States. Foot Ankle Int 2013; 34(11):1486–92.

24. Vakshori V, Sabour AF, Alluri RK, et al. Patient and practice trends in total ankle replacement and tibiotalar arthrodesis in the United States from 2007 to 2013. J Am Acad Orthop Surg 2019;27(2):e77–84.
25. Randsborg PH, Jiang H, Mao J, et al. Two-year revision rates in total ankle replacement versus ankle arthrodesis. J Bone Joint Surg Open Access 2022. https://doi.org/10.2103/JBJS.OA.21.00136. e21.00136.
26. Shih CL, Chen SJ, Huang PJ. Clinical outcomes of total ankle arthroplasty versus ankle arthrodesis for the treatment of end-stage ankle arthritis in the last decade: a systematic review and meta-analysis. J Foot Ankle Surg 2020;59:1032–9.
27. Dannawi Z, Nawabi DH, Patel A, et al. Arthroscopic ankle arthrodesis: are results reproducible irrespective of pre-operative deformity? Foot Ankle Surg 2011;17(4): 294–9.
28. Kim HN, Jeon JY, Noh KC, et al. Arthroscopic ankle arthrodesis with intra-articular distraction. J Foot Ankle Surg 2014;53(4):515–8.
29. Behera S, Patro BP, Das SS, et al. Arthroscopic ankle fusion to manage sequel of loss of lateral malleoli in compound crushed ankle injury. J Clin Orthop Trauma 2019;10(Supple):S231–3.
30. DeVries JG, Hyer CF, Berlet GC. Ankle arthrodesis and malunion takedown to total ankle replacement. In: Roukis TS, Hyer CF, Berlet GC, et al, editors. Primary and revision total ankle replacement: evidence-based surgical management. 2nd edition. Switzerland: Springer Nature; 2021. p. 281–96.
31. Dahl MT, Gulli B, Berg T. Complications of limb lengthening. A learning curve. Clin Orthop Relat Res 1994;301:10–8.
32. Cates NK, Miller JD, Chen S, et al. Safety of tibial half pins with circular external fixation for foot and ankle reconstruction in patients with peripheral neuropathy. J Foot Ankle Surg 2021. https://doi.org/10.1053/j.jfas.2021.12.021. S1067-2516(21)00540-8.

The Ankle Joint
Revision Ankle Fusion Options, Nonunion, Malunion, Protocol for Best Outcome

Nilin M. Rao, DPM, PhD[a],*, Chandler Ligas, DPM[b,c]

KEYWORDS

- Revision • Nonunion • Malunion • Ankle arthrodesis

KEY POINTS

- Evidence shows 100% of nonunions have vitamin D deficiency.
- A specific component in marijuana, tetrahydrocannabinol, has been associated with inhibitory effects of bone metabolism and thus decreased bone mineral density, thus contributing to nonunions.
- When revisional surgery is needed minimal periosteal stripping should be done.
- Duration of surgery, peripheral neuropathy, and A1C greater than 7 are variables that lead to increased complications of nonunion, delayed union, and malunion.
- Contingency management with preoperative carbon monoxide testing to promote smoking cessation efforts can improve compliance and decrease risk of nonunion.

INTRODUCTION

Ankle arthrodesis has been a time-tested procedure for osteoarthritis, avascular necrosis of the talus, deformity correction, and significant trauma of the ankle.[1] Technique guides have created dissection pearls, ease of fixation, and arthroscopic techniques to mitigate complications of the procedure.[2,3] Although advances have been made with the procedure, the potential catastrophic complications of ankle arthrodesis could lead to limb loss. Major complications such as nonunion, malunion, or implant infection are the most worrisome and cumbersome complications to handle. Nonunion rates of ankle arthrodesis range from 2% to 47%; with such a high percentage the management of specific major complications is of paramount importance.[4,5] Therefore, the aim of this article is to provide the practicing surgeon evidence to provide innovative management techniques for nonunion, malunion, and infection following primary ankle arthrodesis.

[a] Foot Specialists of Austin, 1600 West 38th Street, #210, Austin, TX, USA; [b] Podiatric Surgery, Silicon Valley Reconstructive Foot and Ankle Fellowship- Palo Alto Medical Foundation, 701 E El Camino Real 1st Floor, Mountain View, CA 94040, USA; [c] Sunnyvale, CA, USA
* Corresponding author.
E-mail address: raonm1@gmail.com

Clin Podiatr Med Surg 40 (2023) 703–710
https://doi.org/10.1016/j.cpm.2023.05.011
0891-8422/23/© 2023 Elsevier Inc. All rights reserved.
podiatric.theclinics.com

NONUNION

Clinical implications that would suggest that the patient is suffering from a nonunion include progressive pain with ambulation. Clinical findings by the physician would be tenderness of palpation along the arthrodesis site. The defined definition of a nonunion is failure to achieve healing by 9 months with no evidence of progression over the previous 3 months.[6] First-line diagnostic approach to these patients would be serial radiographs; however, standard of care to confirm diagnosis of a nonunion is through computed tomography. Nonunions potentially plaque all arthrodesis procedures of the foot and ankle.[7-9] Nonunions need to be categorized by biologic capacity, deformity, presence or absence of infection, and host status. As others have published, the authors believe that when addressing nonunion revisional surgery, practitioners should take a comprehensive approach to the specific host status of the patient. The authors recommend categorizing host status by risk factor, which can be further broken down into controllable versus uncontrollable. Uncontrollable risk factors include comorbidities of diabetes such as neuropathy, hyperparathyroidism, and growth hormone deficiency, essentially barriers that surgeons cannot change before revisional surgery but should rather optimize through a multiple team approach. Controllable risk factors include smoking, alcohol use, and vitamin D deficiency, essentially any variable that a surgeon can monitor and directly change.

Diabetes and hyperglycemia, both an uncontrollable variable by the surgeon, is well established as a comorbidity causing complications (Source). Although standard of care has been established to prevent elective surgery on patients with an A1c less than 7.[10] Neuropathy is another uncontrollable variable showing evidence linked to complications. O-Connor and colleagues evaluated 82 cases of revisional arthrodesis and evaluated patient factors including diabetes, inflammatory arthropathy, tobacco use, history of infection, nonunion elsewhere, neuropathy, Charcot arthropathy, posttraumatic arthritis, and prior attempt at revision arthrodesis at the same site. Their results showed a statistically significant finding between neuropathy and persistent nonunion.[8] Shibuya and colleagues confirmed these findings when they evaluated 165 diabetic patients who had undergone arthrodesis, osteotomy, or fracture reduction to assess the risk factors associated with nonunion, delayed union, and malunion after elective and nonelective foot and/or ankle surgery. Their results showed bivariant analysis confirming duration of surgery, peripheral neuropathy, and A1C greater than 7 were variables that led to increased complications of nonunion, delayed union, and malunion.[10] One reason the authors believe neuropathy is an associated risk factor is due to patient compliance with non–weight-bearing in the perioperative period. Although operating on patients with neuropathy cannot be avoided in some instances, the surgeons should take additional steps to prevent nonunion development through extensive non–weight-bearing tactics and postoperative management.

Controllable variables that lead to an increased risk of nonunion are smoking, vitamin D deficiency, and substance abuse. Smoking has been associated with negative physiological responses on bone healing and metabolism, specifically speaking about the decreased microperfusion and tissue oxygenation.[11] Patel and colleagues performed a systematic review to elucidate if it was worth discriminating against patients who smoke. Their results specifically found that following ankle arthrodesis in patients who smoke, there was a 3.75 increase in relative risk of nonunions from developing. When controlling all other risk factors, smokers had a 16 times great risk of nonunion.[12] Perlman and colleagues performed a retrospective radiographic review on 88 ankle fusions. Their results had a 28% nonunion rate and found a trend toward significance of nonunion risks factors, which included smoking.[13] Therefore, it is the authors' opinion to completely avoid operating on patients who currently smoke but also to be diligent in contingency management during preoperative evaluation. Certain studies have suggested that smoking cessation 4 weeks before surgery and extending it 4 weeks after surgery can result in an overall decrease in complications, including nonunion.[14] Certain protocols have been established nationally to encourage smoking cessation before surgery but have also provided evidence on preoperative carbon monoxide testing to give practitioners evidence of compliance.[15] Therefore, it is the authors' opinion that if dealt with a patient who has a nonunion and smokes, the surgeon should encourage contingency management with preoperative carbon monoxide testing to promote cessation efforts.

Vitamin D deficiency is another controllable variable that has been linked to risk of developing a nonunion and length of time to union, with some reports suggesting an 8.1 times greater risk of developing nonunion after arthrodesis procedures.[16–18] Most of the evidence in support of supplementation of vitamin D comes from its impact on bone formation and metabolism in healthy individuals.[19] Geographical data show varying amounts of vitamin D deficiency; however, among these groups most (>50%) of their patient populations undergoing foot and ankle surgery have vitamin D deficiency.[20,21] Ramanathan and colleagues evaluated vitamin D deficiency and outcomes after ankle fusion surgery. Their results show that of the patients who underwent reoperation for nonunion, all of their nonunion patients had an associated vitamin D deficiency.[22] Therefore, it is the authors' opinion that when faced with revisional arthrodesis procedures, vitamin D levels should be evaluated. The best test to assess body stores of vitamin D is the 25(OH)D level test, with optimal range of 25 to 80 ng/mL. If deficient, then the authors prefer to supplement the individuals with a loading dose of 50,000 IU and then 1500 to 2000 IU by mouth every day for 4 weeks before surgery.[23,24] The authors will test the individual twice for vitamin D levels before reoperation.

With the increased use of legal marijuana throughout the United States, this specific substance abuse has become more easily studied.[25] Cannabis has been associated with increased risk of revision after total knee arthroplasty and venous thromboemboli.[26,27] A specific component in marijuana, tetrahydrocannabinol, has been associated with inhibitory effects of bone metabolism and thus decreased bone mineral density.[28] Other aspects of the endocannabinoid system (CB1 and CB2) appear from early literature to support healthy bone metabolism and activation of osteoclasts and osteoblasts. Derivatives of the endocannabinoid system maybe more beneficial with patient's perception of pain and chronic pain symptoms as opposed to bone metabolism.[29] Therefore, more evidence needs to be evaluated before the authors can make a definitive answer on the effects of the derivatives from endocannabinoid system; however, the authors encourage cessation of marijuana for all patients before surgery.

Biological capacity of the nonunion is next assessed by the authors. Usually the nature of the nonunion is categorized by hypertrophic, oligotrophic, and atrophic on advanced imaging, and the characteristics of each type allows the surgeons to infer the reason for development of nonunion. Hypertrophic nonunions are the result of instability of the arthrodesis site resulting from high strain at the attempted nonunion.[30] Regardless of the type of hypertrophic nonunion, the optimal treatment of the nonunion is bone stimulation combined with extended periods of non–weight-bearing as a first-line adjuvant.

There are 3 different types of bone stimulators: ultrasound, electrical, and magnetic. Ultrasound-based bone stimulation uses pulses; low-intensity ultrasound is used to stimulate the aggregation and production of certain proteins for useful healing. This is usually done through a transducer on the skin over the nonunion or fracture site. Ultrasound-based bone stimulators are approved through the Food and Drug Administration (FDA) and are termed low-intensity pulsed ultrasound (LIPUS) and low-intensity therapeutic ultrasound (LITUS) (FDA). In a systematic review, LIPUS has been shown to induce micromechanical stress in the arthrodesis site and therefore aid in bone cellular and molecular responses to healing.[31]

Another FDA-approved bone stimulator is the electromagnetic field bone stimulator. There are 3 different types of electromagnetic field bone stimulator, which are capacitive coupling, pulses, and combined magnetic fields. The capacitive coupling is a rather historical approach to bone stimulation placing a stainless steel capacitor plate placed on the skin overlying the nonunion site. Early reports show improved bone nonunion healing up to 77% at an average of 22.5 weeks in a specific case control.[32] However, this approach by itself has fallen out of favor due to clinical studies showing variable safety and efficacy.[33]

The pulsed electromagnetic field bone stimulator is a safe and effective treatment of nonunion of bone by increasing the structural integrity of bone and homeostatic balance.[34] This specific approach has shown to favor graft integration, control the local inflammatory response, and foster tissue repair from both implanted and resident mesenchymal stem cells.[35] Pulsed electromagnetic field bone stimulators have been used in other specialties with increased fusion rates compared with controls.[36] Its use in foot and ankle literature has shown to decrease time to fusion in primary hindfoot arthrodesis and fracture repair in long bones of the foot.[37,38] However, no such studies have evaluated pulsed electromagnetic field bone stimulation on revisional ankle arthrodesis procedures. Nonetheless, it is the authors who recommended adjuvant as first-line therapy for nonunion repair. Manufacturing guidelines suggest its use when the nonunion defect is less than one-half the width of the bone to be treated. The overall treatment duration will vary based on the specific nonunion response to therapy; some suggest its use for 3 to 9 months. The authors will take serial radiographs every month to gauge response.

Combined magnetic fields provide a coil that generates a combination of a static and pulsed magnetic field near the treatment site. Although there is a device approved by the FDA for the use of nonunions, there have been no such reports to show efficacy in foot and ankle literature. Currently, there are only a couple of articles to show favorable outcomes when compared with pulsed electromagnetic field and LIPUS.[39] Therefore, it is the authors' recommendation to avoid this therapy currently.

When the nonunion is unresponsive to bone stimulation and extended non–weight-bearing periods, the surgeon should take the hypertrophic nonunion back for surgical intervention. The goal of the revisional surgery should be to increase mechanical stability; however, practitioners are encouraged at this point to abide by sound surgical principles (AO tenents, Glissan's principles). Of paramount importance is the soft tissue envelope, debridement of the nonunion, to obtain healthy bleeding bone, and then to provide the appropriate fixation. Multiple biomechanical studies have been done to assess the optimal fixation method for ankle arthrodesis.[40–42] Historically the crossing screw configuration was advocated for its ease of use, stability, and resistance against rotational forces.[43] However, to date the anterior locking plate for ankle arthrodesis increases construct stability when supplemented by crossing screw fixation.[44] Therefore, the authors' prefer the supplementation of an anterior plate if not done during the primary ankle fusion.

Atrophic nonunion treatment, after failure of a conservative protocol, is slightly different from the hypertrophic nonunion. Along with the tenets of nonunion repair as discussed previously, the practitioner should pay special attention to the vascularity of the soft tissue envelope; this includes debridement of fibrous tissue, reosteosynthesis, and biological stimulation by bone grafting and growth factor application.[45] Initial planning for the surgery should include the least amount of injury to the soft tissue envelope and should include minimal periosteal stripping. There are a couple of technique pearls that the authors find to be the keys to success. One of these pearls is the use of the Judet technique, which is used to elevate cortical chips that remain attached to the periosteum and overlying soft tissues surrounding the site of nonunion, that when combined with mechanical support leads to bone consolidation.[46] This method has been tested in multiple case series, with radiographic retrospective reviews with greater than 90% boney consolidation following atrophic nonunion repair.[47,48]

As mentioned previously, atrophic nonunion repair should be combined with a growth factor stimulating orthobiologics. Orthobiologics have been well studied for nonunion repair in the lower extremity.[48,49] The authors specifically address the growth factor stimulation with 2 main different modalities. One to provide a scaffold to aid in osteoconductive distribution of osteoblast and one to promote osteoinduction and osteogenesis. When host factors allow, the authors would prefer to use autograft to aid with all 3 of those osteoprogenitor properties. However, because of done site morbidity, the authors prefer to use cancellous chip allograft. It is the authors' opinion that these chips combined with a growth factor stimulating component will act as good as an autograft. For that reason, the authors will combine the cancellous chips with bone marrow aspiration concentration. The growth factor and nonhematopoietic stem cell potential of bone marrow aspirate is well understood.[50,51]

Other orthobiologics have been studied in the literature that also have a place in the atrophic nonunion repair. Mesenchymal stem cells are one such modality that have proved to show great results. Anderson and colleagues reviewed 109 ankle fusions and compared the fusion rate from those with mesenchymal stem cell bone allograft versus proximal tibia autograft. Their results showed no statistically significant different found between the groups and concluded that this mesenchymal stem cell option was comparable with autograft. Currently the authors cannot comment on the viability of platelet-rich plasma, recombinant human platelet derived growth factor (rhPDGF), or other company-sponsored entity usage due to the confounding evidence in the literature. Of note, the authors would like to encourage the readers to evaluate the new literature that is coming out on targeted gene and host progenitor cell therapy for nonunion repair. The evidence shows promising results in stage I clinical trials, and there maybe use for this modality in the near future.

CLINICS CARE POINTS

- Controllable risk (vitamin D, smoking) and uncontrollable risks (diabetes) should be assessed after the diagnosis of ankle nonunion.
- If vitamin D deficient, supplement the individuals with a loading dose of 50,000 IU, then 1500 to 2000 IU by mouth every day for 4 weeks before surgery.
- Further evidence needs to be made for safety and efficacy of marijuana use.
- Atrophic nonunions can be repaired with the Judet technique; periosteal.
- Hypertrophic nonunions should be repaired with bone stimulation and periods of non–weight-bearing before revisional surgery.

DISCLOSURE

None reported.

REFERENCES

1. Albert E. Zur Resektion des Kniegelenkes. Wien Med Press; 1879. p. 20, 705–708.
2. Lindsey BB, Hundal R, Bakshi NK, et al. Ankle arthrodesis through an anterior approach. J Orthop Trauma 2020;34(Suppl 2):S42–3.
3. Hutchinson B. Arthroscopic ankle arthrodesis. Clin Podiatr Med Surg 2016;33(4): 581–9.
4. Overley BD, Rementer MR. Surgical complications of ankle Joint arthrodesis and ankle arthroplasty procedures. Clin Podiatr Med Surg 2017;34(4):565–74. Available at: https://www.sciencedirect.com/science/article/pii/S0891842217300575.
5. Stavrakis AI, SooHoo NF. Trends in complication rates following ankle arthrodesis and total ankle replacement. J Bone Joint Surg Am 2016;98(17):1453–8.
6. Calori GM, Mazza EL, Mazzola S, et al. Non-unions. Clin Cases Miner Bone Metab 2017;14(2):186–8.
7. Klassen LJ, Shi E, Weinraub GM, et al. Comparative nonunion rates in triple arthrodesis. J Foot Ankle Surg 2018;57(6):1154–6.
8. O'Connor KM, Johnson JE, McCormick JJ, et al. Clinical and operative factors related to successful revision arthrodesis in the foot and ankle. Foot Ankle Int 2016;37(8):809–15.
9. Carpenter B. McGlamry's comprehensive textbook of foot and ankle surgery. Philadelphia, PA: Lippincott Williams & Wilkins; 2022.
10. Shibuya N, Humper J, Fluhman B. Factors associated with nonunion, delayed union, and malunion in foot and ankle surgery in diabetic patients. J Foot Ankle Surg 2013;52(2):207–11.
11. Lee JJ, Patel R, Biermann JS, et al. The musculoskeletal effects of cigarette smoking. J Bone Joint Surg Am 2013;95:850–9.
12. Kim JH, Patel S. Is it worth discriminating against patients who smoke? A systematic literature review on the effects of tobacco use in foot and ankle surgery. J Foot Ankle Surg 2017;56(3):594–9.
13. Perlman M, Thordarson D. Ankle fusion in a high risk population: an assessment of nonunion risk factors. Foot Ankle Int 1999;20:491–6.
14. Lindstrom DL, Sadr Azodi OS, Wladis A, et al. Effects of a perioperative smoking cessation intervention on postoperative complications: a randomized trial. Ann Surg 2008;248:739–45.
15. Dallery J, Raiff BR, Kim SJ, et al. Nationwide access to an internet-based contingency management intervention to promote smoking cessation: a randomized controlled trial. Addiction 2017;112(5):875–83.
16. Smith JT, Halim K, Palms DA, et al. Prevalence of vitamin D deficiency in patients with foot and ankle injuries. Foot Ankle Int 2014;35:8–13.
17. Ravindra VM, Godzik J, Dailey AT, et al. Vitamin D levels and 1-year fusion outcomes in elective spine surgery: a prospective observational study. Spine (Phila Pa 1976) 2015;40:1536–41.
18. Moore KR, Howell MA, Saltrick KR, et al. Risk factors associated with nonunion after elective foot and ankle reconstruction: a case-control study. J Foot Ankle Surg 2017;56(3):457–62.
19. Eschle D, Aeschlimann AG. Is supplementation of vitamin D beneficial for fracture healing? A short review of the literature. Geriatr Orthop Surg Rehabil 2011;2:90–3.

20. Aujla RS, Allen PE, Ribbans WJ. Vitamin D levels in 577 consecutive elective foot & ankle surgery patients. Foot Ankle Surg 2019;25(3):310–5.
21. Michelson JD, Charlson MD. Vitamin D status in an elective orthopedic surgical population. Foot Ankle Int 2016;37(2):186–91.
22. Ramanathan D, Emara AK, Pinney S, et al. Vitamin D deficiency and outcomes after ankle fusion: a short report. Foot Ankle Int 2022;43(5):703–5.
23. Kennel KA, Drake MT, Hurley DL. Vitamin D deficiency in adults: When to test and how to treat. Mayo Clinic proceedings 2010;85(8):752–8.
24. Substance Abuse Center for Behavioral Health Statistics and Quality. Results from the 2018 national survey on drug use and health: detailed tables. Rockville, MD: SAMHSA; 2020. Accessed January 6, 2022.
25. Sophocleous A, Robertson R, Ferreira NB, et al. Heavy cannabis use is associated with low bone mineral density and an increased risk of fractures. Am J Med 2017;130(2):214–21.
26. Law TY, Kurowicki J, Rosas S, et al. Cannabis use increases risk for revision after total knee arthroplasty. J Long Term Eff Med Implants 2018;28(2):125–30.
27. Vakharia RM, Sodhi N, Anis HK, et al. Patients who have cannabis use disorder have higher rates of venous thromboemboli, readmission rates, and costs following primary total knee arthroplasty. J Arthroplasty 2020;35(4):997–1002.
28. Heath D, Koslosky E, Bartush K, et al. Marijuana in orthopaedics: effects on bone health, wound-healing, surgical complications, and pain management. JBJS Reviews 2022;10(2). https://doi.org/10.2106/JBJS.RVW.21.00184.
29. White CM. A review of human studies assessing cannabidiol's (CBD) therapeutic actions and potential. J Clin Pharmacol 2019;59(7):923–34.
30. Gatti A, Tarantino U, Gasparini M, et al. Locking screw augmentation in hypertrophic nonunion of tibia: a novel surgical technique. Acta Biomed 2021;92(S1):e2021434.
31. Mundi R, Petis S, Kaloty R, et al. Low-intensity pulsed ultrasound: fracture healing. Indian J Orthop 2009;43(2):132–40.
32. Brighton CT, Pollack SR. Treatment of recalcitrant non-union with a capacitively coupled electrical field. A preliminary report. JBJS 1985;67(4):577–85.
33. Griffin XL, Costa ML, Parsons N, et al. Electromagnetic field stimulation for treating delayed union or non-union of long bone fractures in adults. Cochrane Database Syst Rev 2011;(4):CD008471.
34. Cadossi R, Massari L, Racine-Avila J, et al. Pulsed electromagnetic field stimulation of bone healing and Joint preservation: cellular mechanisms of skeletal response. J Am Acad Orthop Surg Glob Res Rev 2020;4(5):e1900155.
35. Varani K, Vincenzi F, Pasquini S, et al. Pulsed electromagnetic field stimulation in osteogenesis and chondrogenesis: signaling pathways and therapeutic implications. Int J Mol Sci 2021;22(2):809.
36. Foley K. Randomized, prospective, and controlled clinical trial of pulsed electromagnetic field Page 22 of 23 stimulation for cervical fusion. Spine J 2008;8(3):436–42.
37. Dhawan SK, Conti SF, Towers J. The effect of pulsed electromagnetic fields on hindfoot arthrodesis: a prospective study. J Foot Ankle Surg 2004;43(2):93–6.
38. Streit A. Effect on clinical outcome and growth factor synthesis with adjunctive use of pulsed electromagnetic fields for fifth metatarsal nonunion fracture: a double-blind randomized study. Ankle Int 2016;37(9):919–23.
39. Cheaney B 2nd, El Hashemi M, Obayashi J, et al. Combined magnetic field results in higher fusion rates than pulsed electromagnetic field bone stimulation after thoracolumbar fusion surgery. J Clin Neurosci 2020;74:115–9.

40. Dohm MP, Benjamin JB, Harrison J, et al. A biomechanical evaluation of three forms of internal fixation used in ankle arthrodesis. Foot Ankle Int 1994;15(6): 297–300.
41. Somberg AM, Whiteside WK, Nilssen E, et al. Biomechanical evaluation of a second generation headless compression screw for ankle arthrodesis in a cadaver model. Foot Ankle Surg 2016;22(1):50–4.
42. Wang S, Yu J, Ma X, et al. Finite element analysis of the initial stability of arthroscopic ankle arthrodesis with three-screw fixation: posteromedial versus posterolateral home-run screw. J Orthop Surg Res 2020;15(1):252.
43. Nasson S, Shuff C, Palmer D, et al. Biomechanical comparison of ankle arthrodesis techniques: crossed screws vs. blade plate. Foot Ankle Int 2001;22(7): 575–80.
44. Tarkin IS, Mormino MA, Clare MP, et al. Anterior plate supplementation increases ankle arthrodesis construct rigidity. Foot Ankle Int 2007;28(2):219–23.
45. Rupp M, Kern S, El Khassawna T, et al. Do systemic factors influence the fate of nonunions to become atrophic? A retrospective analysis of 162 cases. BioMed Res Int 2019;2019:6407098.
46. Judet PR, Patel A. Muscle pedicle bone grafting of long bones by osteoperiosteal decortication. Clin Orthop Relat Res 1972;87:74–80.
47. Guyver P, Wakeling C, Naik K, et al. Judet osteoperiosteal decortication for treatment of non-union: the Cornwall experience. Injury 2012;43(7):1187–92.
48. Cho Y, Byun YS, Suh JD, et al. Osteoperiosteal decortication and autogenous cancellous bone graft combined with bridge plating for non-hypertrophic diaphyseal nonunion. Clin Orthop Surg 2021;13(3):301–6.
49. Malhotra R, Kumar V, Garg B, et al. Role of autologous platelet-rich plasma in treatment of long-bone nonunions: a prospective study. Musculoskelet Surg 2015;99(3):243–8.
50. Schäfer R, DeBaun MR, Fleck E, et al. Quantitation of progenitor cell populations and growth factors after bone marrow aspirate concentration. J Transl Med 2019; 17(1):115.
51. Shapiro G, Lieber R, Gazit D, et al. Recent advances and future of gene therapy for bone regeneration. Curr Osteoporos Rep 2018;16(4):504–11.

The Ankle Joint

Management of Significant Bone Loss with Arthrodesis

Helene R. Cook, DPM, AACFAS[a], Garret Strand, DPM, AACFAS[a],
Collin Messerly, DPM, AACFAS[b], Jason Nowak, DPM, FACFAS[a],*

KEYWORDS

- Arthrodesis • Tibiocalcaneal arthrodesis • Femoral head allograft • Bone graft
- Talar allograft • Titanium cage • Truss

KEY POINTS

- Surgical management of significant bone loss of the ankle joint warrants a comprehensive approach to patient care including evaluation, imaging, and preoperative planning.
- Primary goals include pain relief, deformity correction, preservation of limb length, as well as a stable hindfoot and ankle complex.
- Decisions on approach and fixation constructs are based on deformity, earlier surgical procedures, and existing hardware.
- Patient education on postoperative expectations and potential complications is crucial to surgical outcomes.

INTRODUCTION

Segmental bone loss of the tibia and/or talus presents a challenge for the foot and ankle surgeon. Bone loss at the level of the ankle joint can be due to several causes. These include failed total ankle arthroplasty, tibiotalar nonunion, talar avascular necrosis, Charcot neuroarthropathy, bone tumors, infection, and trauma.[1,2] Only a few viable surgical treatment options have been described to reconstruct bony height, and oftentimes, these serve as the only alternative to a below-the-knee amputation. From a review of the literature, these surgical interventions include bone transport with external fixation, vascularized autograft transfer, bulk frozen and fresh allograft, bulk autograft spacers, tibiotalocalcaneal (TTC) arthrodesis, tibiocalcaneal (TC) arthrodesis, distal tibial lengthening, or a combination of the above.[2] During the past decade, there has been an increase in the number of surgeons adopting these techniques in addition to an increase in the various fixation construct options. However, the published research

[a] Shasta Orthopaedics and Sports Medicine, 1255 Liberty Street, Redding, CA 96001, USA;
[b] Town Center Orthopedics, 44095 Pipeline Plaza, Suite 370, Ashburn, VA 20147, USA
* Corresponding author.
E-mail address: norcalrfaf@gmail.com

Clin Podiatr Med Surg 40 (2023) 711–724
https://doi.org/10.1016/j.cpm.2023.05.012
0891-8422/23/© 2023 Elsevier Inc. All rights reserved.

podiatric.theclinics.com

on these various techniques remains limited to case reports and small case series without much documented long-term follow-up outcomes. Regardless of the cause, the primary goals of surgical correction are to restore limb length as well as to achieve a painless, stable, plantigrade foot. Successfully achieving this will reduce physical disability and limit the need for external shoe modifications and bracing requirements.

DISCUSSION OF VARIOUS SURGICAL MANAGEMENT OPTIONS AND THEIR REPORTED OUTCOMES
Fibular Autograft

There have been a couple recent reports detailing the use of fibular autograft to reconstruct large bony defects at the ankle joint.

One such study by Watanabe and colleagues[3] reported an arthrodesis procedure using soft tissue-preserved fibular graft to maintain limb length. The authors detail an anterolateral approach to the ankle performing a transverse osteotomy of the fibula. They maintained both lateral and posterior skin and soft tissue aspects of the transected fibula. The patient's nonviable talus was resected with the preservation of the talar head and neck if possible. The cartilaginous surfaces of the distal tibia and dorsal calcaneus were prepared for fusion, and the transected fibular was either used as a strut graft in combination with iliac bone graft or made into 2 segments to fill the bony defect. Their preferred fixation method was the use of an intramedullary nail and 4.0 cancellous screws to fixate the fibular to the lateral aspect of tibia and calcaneus. Postoperatively, they required patients to be non–weight-bearing for 4 weeks and progressing to full weight-bearing by the eighth week. All of the patients in their study had boney fusion by 3 months. They found that their American Orthopaedic Foot & Ankle Society (AOFAS) score before reconstructive intervention was 53.8 and improved to 75.5 at the time of final follow-up. The advantages to their procedural technique include ease of access and a wide view of the ankle. Additionally, the use of a fibular strut autograft is thought to restore the blood supply and preserve lower extremity height.[3]

More recently, Bernasconi and colleagues[4] described a similar technique using fibular pillar autografting. They utilized a distal lateral approach and then performed an oblique fibular cut about 8 to 12 cm from the tip of the fibula. The distal tibial and calcaneal articular surfaces were prepared for arthrodesis and the resected fibula was sectioned into either 3 or 4 columns depending on the height of the graft required to fill the articular gap. If necessary, they harvested iliac crest autograft to augment. Their preferred fixation constructs to stabilize their graft were either intramedullary locking nail fixation or lateral locking plates. Postoperatively, they kept their patients non–weight-bearing for 6 weeks and then gradual progression to full weight-bearing by 8 to 12 weeks. In their cohort, 83% of patients achieved union and were satisfied with their outcomes.[4]

The use of autograft has its well-known advantages in bone substitution because it provides the body's natural osteogenic cells and associated growth factors. Autograft also is readily available, has no risk of disease transmission, and is low-cost relative to other graft types. These grafts do not come without the risk of donor site morbidity such as wound complications, fractures, and donor site pain.[1,5] Additionally, autograft from places such as the fibula or iliac crest is limited in the amount harvested so as to not compromise the stability of the donor site.

Fresh Bulk Talar Allograft

The use of fresh-frozen bulk talar allograft is rare upon literature review but was most recently described by DeFontes and colleagues.[6] Indications for their use of bulk talar allograft include avascular necrosis of the talus and posttraumatic collapse of the talus in patients with a preserved soft tissue envelope and viable talar head and neck (**Fig. 1**). Contraindications for their specific technique included candidates in which the whole talus was involved including the head and neck or those with active infection, tobacco use, and uncontrolled diabetes. Their technique allows for the preservation of a viable talar neck not only for its bone stock but also for its blood supply. They propose that the allograft talus may be better suited biomechanically to accommodate the compressive forces at the ankle joint than that of an allograft femoral head allograft (FHA) due to the orientation of trabecular bone.[6]

Their operative technique included a lateral approach to the ankle joint with fibular resection. The resected fibula was milled for additional bone graft at the arthrodesis sites. The nonviable talar bone was excised with careful dissection to maintain any remaining vascular attachments to the healthy talar neck and head. The remaining distal tibial and dorsal calcaneal surfaces were then prepared for arthrodesis. A fresh frozen laterality matched talus was also denuded of cartilage at its dorsal and plantar articulations. They then recommend soaking the talar allograft in autologous aspirate before implantation. DeFontes and colleagues used a combination of fixation including an intramedullary hindfoot nail and compression screws across the native talus into the graft talus (**Fig. 2**). Postoperatively their patients were to be non–weight-bearing for 12 weeks with a goal of full weight-bearing at 16 weeks.[6,7]

This group further published a small case series on the outcomes of their patients who underwent fresh bulk talar allograft.[7] Although this study had a small cohort, their results show a 100% fusion rate with the mean time to fusion being 7.2 months. They reported minimal complications with no infections and one removal of hardware due to proximal stress reaction and pain. They reported no graft collapse and their patients reported improvements in multiple functional outcome measurements at 12 months follow-up.[7]

The use of allograft is advantageous in that some types of bulk allograft are readily available, their size is not limited, and they are resistant to compressive forces. However, allograft spacers do come with the risk of disease transmission, higher costs, and some types of allografts are limited by donor availability.[6]

Bulk Femoral Head Allograft

One of the most studied and recognized procedures during the last couple of decades for restoring bony height is the use of a femoral head allograft (FHA). This large bone

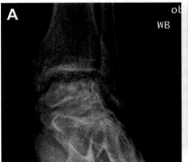
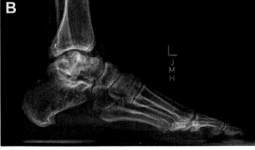

Fig. 1. (*A*) Anteroposterior and (*B*) lateral preoperative radiographs demonstrate patient with talar osteonecrosis. (Original Figures/Tables using previously published data: "Data from Vaughn J, DeFontes KW 3rd, Keyser C, Bluman EM, Smith JT. Case Series: Allograft Tibiotalocalcaneal Arthrodesis Utilizing Fresh Talus. Foot Ankle Orthop. 2019;4(2):2473011419834541.")

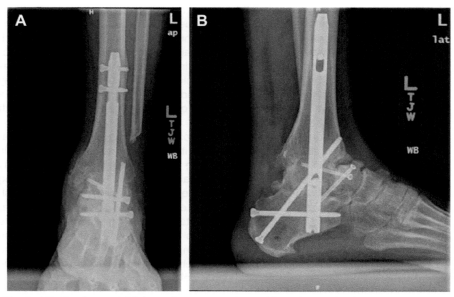

Fig. 2. (*A*) Mortice and (*B*) lateral postoperative ankle radiographs demonstrating graft incorporation and TTC arthrodesis. (Original Figures/Tables using previously published data: "Data from Vaughn J, DeFontes KW 3rd, Keyser C, Bluman EM, Smith JT. Case Series: Allograft Tibiotalocalcaneal Arthrodesis Utilizing Fresh Talus. Foot Ankle Orthop. 2019;4(2):2473011419834541.")

block allograft has proven to be readily available in most hospital facilities and is thought to meet the structural demands of the ankle joint. Both its volume and cortico-canellous structure are able to replace large voids, restore height to the joint, and with-stand reaming for intramedullary fixation.[8] There are various studies detailing their outcomes as well as various technical approaches.

A number of earlier reports described high nonunion rates and poor clinical outcomes for the use of FHA. Fusion rates in the literature have fluctuated between 45% and 90% with a high incidence of graft collapse.[9,10] Jeng and colleagues reported a 71% rate in functional limb salvage with a 50% rate of radiographic fusion. In a study by Bussewitz and colleagues, they reviewed 25 patients who had undergone an FHA with intramedul-lary nail fixation. They found that 21 of 25 (84%) were deemed successful. Of these 21, only 12 were reported as clinical unions giving a 48% fusion rate.[11] Berkowitz and col-leagues achieved a 66.7% fusion rate with FHA and intramedullary nailing in patients presenting with failed total ankle arthroplasty (TAA). Interestingly, all of their nonunions occurred at the subtalar joint. The amputation rates of 2 of the earlier 2 studies, Jeng and colleagues[10] and Buzzewitz and colleagues,[11] were 16% and 19%, respectively. These rates of amputation are not dissimilar to the rates of amputation following tibiotalarcal-caneal (TTC) arthrodesis without complex bony voids. The amputation rate following TTC arthrodesis without the use of grafts has been reported to range from 2% to 17%.[12] One of the other disadvantages of bulk FHA that has been described is graft subsidence or collapse. In a recent study by Steele and colleagues,[8] they found that 4 out of 7 or 57.1% had graft resorption.

Rogero and colleagues demonstrated a rate of radiographic union at both the ankle and subtalar joint was 63%, and their rate of one joint fusion was 88%. However, when they combined radiographic unions with clinically functional limb salvage, their success rate was 88% or 21 of 24 limbs.[13] Their complication rate was 29%, which included 3 nonunions requiring revisional procedures. They reported a 0% rate of lower leg amputation.[13] Overall, this study supported the use of FHA and intramedullary nail fixation as a respectable method for large bony defects at the ankle joint.

Additionally, Coetzee and colleagues recently published a retrospective review of 45 patients who had undergone hindfoot fusion using FHA. Their results ultimately support the use of these FHAs to improve significantly patients' pain and function. They also reported a high average rate of fusion at 90% for both ankle and TCarthrodesis with FHA.[9] They think that an important reason for their high fusion rates had to do with their described technique. For their TC arthrodesis with FHA, they used a transfibular approach with the resection of the distal fibula. They used acetabular cup and cone reamers to create congruent fusion surfaces for the FHA. This group used rigid internal fixation and incorporated a bridge graft to provide support while the FHA incorporated. The bridge graft functions to give the construct rotational, bending, and axial stability. They reported 5 nonunions of which all of them, their bridge graft did not heal.[9]

Haong and colleagues detail their surgical technique for TC arthrodesis with FHA using a cup and cone acetabular reamer similar to that described by Cuttica and colleagues. They obtained bone marrow aspirate (BMA) from the proximal tibia, which was concentrated and later used to soak their FHA. They describe a lateral approach to the ankle with the resection of the distal fibula. Other authors such as Coeztee, ground the distal fibula in a bone mill to be used as further autograft in their construct.[9] Then the remaining talus and all other devitalized bone were removed. They then used cone-shaped acetabular reamers measuring 34 and 39 mm to ream the distal tibia and dorsal calcaneus with the goal of creating a concentric area to accept the FHA.[14,15] These surfaces were then fenestrated to prepare for the graft. Next, the FHA was prepared using the same-sized cup-shaped acetabular reamer to make sure the graft had as much contact area with the patient's native bone as possible. They then used a large diameter guidewire to fenestrate the femoral head surface and soaked it in the previously made BMA. They then introduced the FHA and proceeded with the placement of an intramedullary nail.[14,15] They advocate for the addition of two 4.5-mm cannulated screws to compress the remaining talar head to the FHA. Haong and colleagues keep these patients non–weight-bearing for 10 to 12 weeks followed by transitioning into a cam walker boot for an additional 2 to 3 months.

Titanium Cages

Instead of relying on bony allografts and autografts, there have been multiple reports on the use of titanium cages in the arthrodesis of ankle and hindfoot salvage procedures.

Palmanovich and colleagues describe the use of cylindrical titanium spinal cages filled with local bone graft to provide a stable, well-aligned fusion. One of the main advantages to using a spinal cage is that it is readily available in multiple sizes on the shelf of most major hospital facilities because it is generally indicated for spinal fusion procedures. Their technique includes the preparation of articulation areas, the application of spinal titanium mesh cage filled with morselized cancellous bone autograft/allograft in the area of defect fixated by either intramedullary fixation or titanium screw/plate fixation. Postoperatively, they kept their patients non–weight-bearing for 12 weeks until fusion was observed. They observed complete union in all 7 of their patient cohort within 6 to 12 months postoperatively and only 2 complications that were resolved. They describe the relative safety of this technique as well as the ability to effectively maintain mechanical stability and appropriate lower extremity length.[16]

Additionally, there have been a handful of reports on the use of 3-D titanium truss cages for bony defects of the hindfoot and ankle. Preston and colleagues detail the use of a 3-D printed cage to salvage a failed total ankle replacement. They were able to use the original anterior ankle incision to remove the original hardware and implant a custom titanium truss cage with a mixture of autologous and autologous graft. They were able to design the custom cage to allow for intramedullary nail fixation. Even though their study was limited to a single patient, their patient went on to heal uneventfully, and at 1 year postoperatively continued to be able to fully ambulate pain free in normal shoe gear.[17] A small number of studies also reported on the use of titanium cages for salvage attempts after severe ankle trauma. Both reports went onto successful TTC arthrodesis, and the patients were able to ambulate as well as work independently at their 1-year follow-up.[18,19]

Bejarano-Pineda and colleagues described their clinic outcomes and radiographic union rates for a case series of 7 patients who underwent hindfoot arthrodesis with use of custom 3-D cage and intramedullary nail fixation. Six of their patients were reported to have greater than 50% bony bridging with a mean time to union of 9.8 months.[1] Ultimately, they concluded that in a patient population that is at risk of nonunions, the use of titanium cages and intramedullary nail fixation allows for an optimal alternative with high rates of union.

Further, Steele and colleagues[20] recently compared their use of TC arthrodesis with FHA to those of 3-D printed titanium spherical cages. They found that the rate of total fused articulation was significantly higher in the 3-D cage group than that of the FHA group with a rate of 92% and 62%, respectively. The number of patients who had successful fusion of all 3 articulations (tibia, calcaneus, and talar neck) was also higher in the 3-D group with 75% compared with that of the allograft group at 42.9%.[20] Overall, they supported the use of 3D custom spherical cages as a safe and successful alternative in addressing these complex hindfoot and ankle patients (**Figs. 3–5**).

The use of titanium cages in hindfoot fusions with segmental bone defects allows for not only structural support but also maintenance of limb length.[21,22] These implants offer a strong scaffold for bone incorporation. One of the major advantages of using

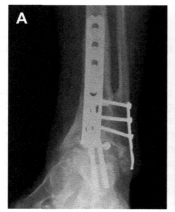
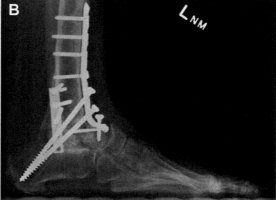

Fig. 3. (*A*) Mortice and (*B*) lateral preoperative radiographs demonstrating patients failed femoral bone block after previously failed total ankle replacement.

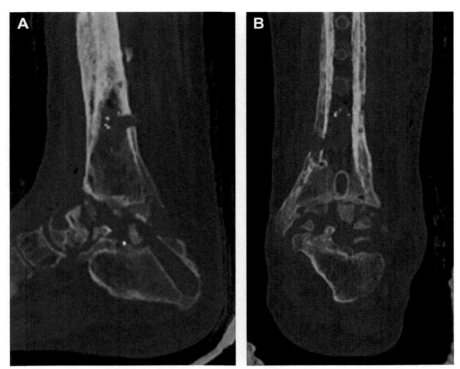

Fig. 4. (*A*) Sagittal and (*B*) coronal MRI demonstrating avascular necrosis of femoral bone block and cystic changes.

a titanium cage whether it be a spinal cage or a 3-D custom implant is that it mitigates the need for large donor site morbidity to obtain sizable autograft as well as prevents any bone graft migration or subsidence.[1,2,16,17,21] The disadvantage to these cages is that they are not inherently osteoinductive, angiogenic, and osteogenic; however, they do allow for the concomitant use of allograft or autograft to potentiate union rates.

With the recent advances in technology and increase in availability to 3-D printing, custom cages can be designed to patient-specific defects. This innovative technology can also create designs to allow for deformity correction as well. The designs have roughened titanium surfaces to allow for maximum bony bridging, fusion, and increased fit between implant and bone interface.[1,2,20–22] The overall cost of these procedures and using customized technology, unfortunately still remains high and may serve as the biggest limitation for use.

POTENTIAL COMPLICATIONS

For all the surgical procedures offered above, general complications include damage to the various nerves and vessels surrounding the ankle, venous thromboembolism, delayed wound healing, nonunion, malunion, deep infection, superficial infection, a need for further surgery, and proximal amputation.

Depending on the approach to the ankle, the superficial and deep peroneal nerves, sural nerve, and posterior tibial nerves are all at risk. We recommend careful dissection and appropriate retraction to minimize this risk throughout the case. Additionally, we

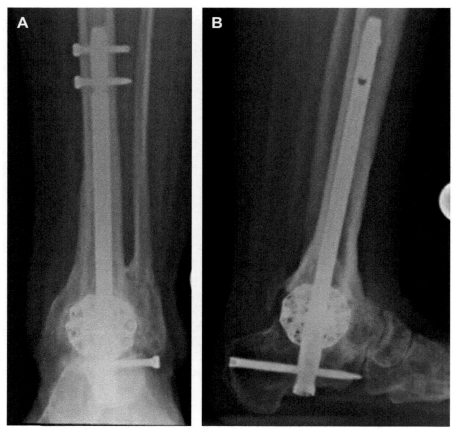

Fig. 5. (A) Anteroposterior and (B) lateral 6-year postoperative radiographs demonstrating union and incorporation through the titanium cage.

highly recommend preoperative risk stratification for venous thromboembolism and the use of a combination of chemoprophylaxis and mechanoprophylaxis intraoperatively and postoperatively while the patient is non–weight-bearing.

Because this is likely not the patient's index procedure, the surgeon is likely to encounter scar tissue from previous procedures. Additionally, these patients tend to be immunocompromised or dealing with multiple other comorbidities. Therefore, due to the nature of these cases, the potential for superficial and deep infection is significant. We recommend appropriate preoperative, intraoperative, and postoperative antibiotic use as well as a tension free closure through a multi-layered approach.

One of the most devastating complications is the chance of a nonunion. In order to prevent nonunions, we recommend thorough joint preparation, maximizing the host bone to allograft bone/cage contact, and rigid internal fixation. Further, we encourage any techniques that allow for the incorporation of additional autograft or allograft substitutes. If possible, autograft is preferred through the forms of milled bone, BMA, or harvesting from a site far from the fusion areas. Autograft bone provides osteoconductive, osteogenic, and osteoinductive properties, whereas allograft bone only has an osteoconductive role.[23]

As these procedures are generally final salvage attempts, in the case of severe complication, below-the-knee amputation may be required, and patients should be appropriately educated on this in the preoperative period.

CASE STUDY

A 59-year-old man with a past medical history of bilateral total ankle arthroplasties presented to the senior author's (J.N.) clinic with complaints of pain and inability to ambulate on his right side. Unfortunately, his left total ankle arthroplasty previously failed and he elected for a left below-the-knee amputation. Clinical examination and preoperative imaging of his right ankle showed a complete dislocation of the talar component, a fractured medial malleolus, and significant instability of the ankle joint (**Figs. 6** and **7**). After lengthy discussion about the patient's conservative and surgical options, the patient elected for limb salvage attempts.

The patient was brought to the operating room for explantation of total ankle prosthesis, distal fibular autograft harvest, and TC arthrodesis with FHA and intramedullary fixation.

Patient positioning is critical to the success and maximal surgical efficiency. For this patient, we proceeded with a supine approach, making sure to adequately bump the ipsilateral hip so that the foot sits neutral and not externally or internally rotated to the leg. It is important to also provide a sterile bump under the distal tibia during the procedure to allow the foot to rest neutral to the tibia and not displaced either anterior or posterior. Furthermore, we place the heel slightly off the bed to assist with ease of reduction and positioning however dependent on the fixation construct this may not be necessary.

We advocate a transfibular approach for this patient to allow for harvesting of the distal fibula for autograft as well as adequate access to the ankle joint for the removal of implant. The distal third of the fibula was resected, soft tissue and cartilage was removed, and the bone was placed in a bone mill to produce autograft. We will also take autograft from a site such as the proximal tibia, distal tibia, or calcaneus if it is

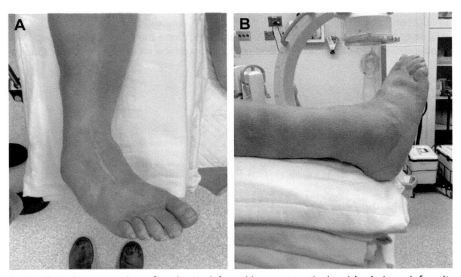

Fig. 6. Clinical presentation of patient's right ankle preoperatively with obvious deformity.

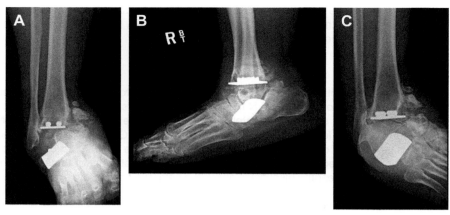

Fig. 7. (A) Anteroposterior, (B) lateral, and (C) mortice preoperative radiographs demonstrating patient's subluxed implant and signifiant ankle deformity.

feasible to augment our arthrodesis site. The implant was then accessed and removed without any evidence of infection (**Figs. 8** and **9**). If, at this time, there is a concern for infection, frozen sections can be quickly prepared and analyzed by a pathologist before proceeding with the case. Additionally, the nonviable remaining talus was removed. If it is possible, the senior author tries to keep the talar head and neck; however, in this case, neither were viable, and the talus was removed in total.

At this time, we then advocate for a very thorough preparation of the arthrodesis sites. In this case, we elected to use acetabular reamers to remove any remaining cartilage from the distal tibia, dorsal calcaneus. Any autograft we could save from the reaming we put aside to later augment. The matching acetabular cup reamer was used to also denude the bulk FHA of its cartilage. Utilizing the acetabular cup and cone reamers in our opinion allows for a better bone-on-bone interface and increased contact surface area between the two. We also fenestrate all the surfaces, and drill channels through the femoral head to further increase the surface area. This is all augmented with autograft.

Concerning positioning of the FHA in this case, since the talar head and neck were removed, we made sure the FHA and navicular interface were well matched. Once we

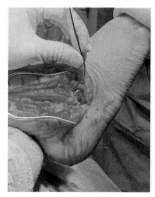
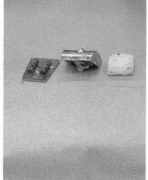
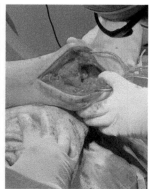

Fig. 8. Resection of fibula and removal of existing implant.

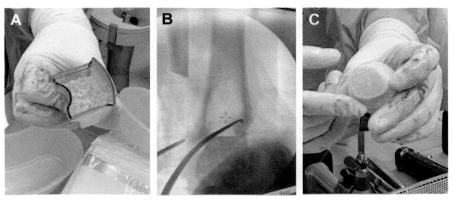

Fig. 9. (A) Milled fibular autograft, (B) fluoroscopic image of defect, and (C) femoral head allograft.

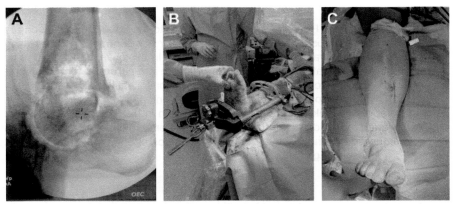

Fig. 10. (A) Fluoroscopic image of ankle with FHA, (B) intraoperative image of intramedullary nail implantation, and (C) postoperative clinical image showing reduction of original deformity.

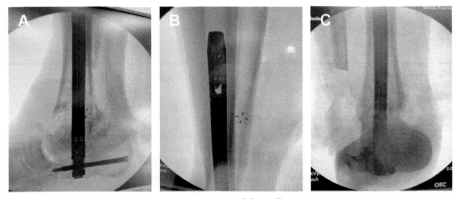

Fig. 11. (A, B) Lateral and (C) anteroposterior of final fluoroscopy images.

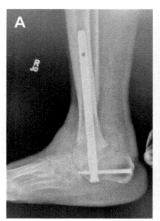
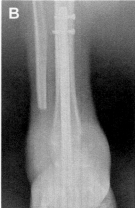
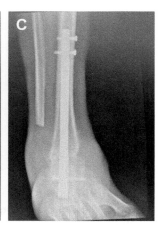

Fig. 12. (*A*) Anteroposterior, (*B*) lateral, and (*C*) mortice radiographs demonstrating graft incorporation and TTC arthrodesis.

liked the location of our FHA and the foot sat neutral to the tibia with the second ray inline to the tibial tuberosity, we temporarily fixed our position making sure to keep this fixation out of the way of our permanent fixation. In this case, we elected to use an intramedullary nail fixation device that provides both internal and external compression over time to allow for the best chance at bony consolidation (**Figs. 10** and **11**).

Postoperatively, the patient was placed in a splint and remained non–weight-bearing for about 6 weeks. There is notable reduction in his deformity with a rectus and well-aligned foot underneath the tibia. Patient seems to have graft incorporation and bony consolidation now at more than 6 months postoperatively and continues to be monitored closely (**Fig. 12**).

SUMMARY

Significant bone loss at the level of the ankle joint is a devastating and painful condition, which can greatly limit a patient's functional capacity. When conservative measures have been exhausted, surgery is an option. Operative treatment of these deformities is not only technically challenging but also the outcomes have been shown to be less predictable compared with surgical treatment of other conditions in the foot and ankle.

CLINICS CARE POINTS

- Segmental bone loss of the distal tibia and/or talus presents a challenge to successful reconstruction for the foot and ankle surgeon.
- Current treatment options to defects at the ankle joint include bone transport, bulk allografts, bulk autografts, titanium cages, and external fixation techniques.
- Unfortunately, these procedures are generally a final salvage attempt and based on the limited amount of current literature, a substantial number of patients are left with a chronically painful extremity or require proximal amputation.
- As the continued use of these techniques increases, larger cohorts of patients should be studied to improve surgical outcomes and techniques.

FINANCIAL DISCLOSURES

H.R. Cook, DPM, AACFAS; C. Messerly, DPM, AACFAS: have no financial disclosures, commercial associations, or any other conditions posing a conflict of interest to report. Garret Strand, DPM, AACFAS reports he is a consultant for Redpoint and Enovis/DJO. J. Nowak, DPM, FACFAS reports he is a consultant for Redpoint and Enovis/DJO.

ACKNOWLEDGMENTS

The authors would like to thank Samuel Adams, MD for his contributions to the clinical case figures within this publication. This article was supported by Shasta Orthopedics & Sports Medicine.

REFERENCES

1. Bejarano-Pineda L, Sharma A, Adams SB, et al. Three-dimensional printed cage in patients with tibiotalocalcaneal arthrodesis using a retrograde intramedullary nail: early outcomes. Foot Ankle Spec 2021;14(5):401–9.
2. Abar B, Kwon N, Allen NB, et al. Outcomes of surgical reconstruction using custom 3D-printed porous titanium implants for critical-sized bone defects of the foot and ankle. Foot Ankle Int 2022;43(6):750–61.
3. Watanabe K, Teramoto A, Kobayashi T, et al. Tibiotalocalcaneal arthrodesis using a soft tissue-preserved fibular graft for treatment of large bone defects in the ankle. Foot Ankle Int 2017;38(6):671–6.
4. Bernasconi A, Patel S, Malhotra K, et al. Salvage tibiotalocalcaneal arthrodesis augmented with fibular columns and iliac crest autograft: a technical note. Foot Ankle Spec 2021;14(1):79–88.
5. Berkowitz MJ, Clare MP, Walling AK, et al. Salvage of failed total ankle arthroplasty with fusion using structural allograft and internal fixation. Foot Ankle Int 2011;32:S493–502.
6. DeFontes KW 3rd, Vaughn J, Smith J, et al. Tibiotalocalcaneal arthrodesis with bulk talar allograft for treatment of talar osteonecrosis. Foot Ankle Int 2018; 39(4):506–14.
7. Vaughn J, DeFontes KW 3rd, Keyser C, et al. Case series: allograft tibiotalocalcaneal arthrodesis utilizing fresh talus. Foot Ankle Orthop 2019;4(2). 2473011419834541.
8. Steele JR, Lazarides AL, DeOrio JK. Tibiotalocalcaneal arthrodesis using a novel retrograde intramedullary nail. Foot Ankle Spec 2020;13(6):463–9.
9. Coetzee JC, Den Hartog BD, Stone McGaver R, et al. Femoral head allografts for talar body defects. Foot Ankle Int 2021;42(7):815–23.
10. Jeng CL, Campbell JT, Tang EY, et al. Tibiotalocalcaneal arthrodesis with bulk femoral head allograft for salvage of large defects in the ankle. Foot Ankle Int 2013;34(9):1256–66.
11. Bussewitz B, DeVries JG, Dujela M, et al. Retrograde intramedullary nail with femoral head allograft for large deficit tibiotalocalcaneal arthrodesis. Foot Ankle Int 2014;35(7):706–11.
12. Lee BH, Fang C, Kunnasegaran R, et al. Tibiotalocalcaneal arthrodesis with the hindfoot arthrodesis nail: a prospective consecutive series from a single institution. J Foot Ankle Surg 2018;57:23–30.
13. Rogero R, Tsai J, Fuchs D, et al. Midterm results of radiographic and functional outcomes after tibiotalocalcaneal arthrodesis with bulk femoral head allograft. Foot Ankle Spec 2020;13(4):315–23.

14. Cuttica DJ, Hyer CF. Femoral head allograft for tibiotalocalcaneal fusion using a cup and cone reamer technique. J Foot Ankle Surg 2011;50:126–9.
15. Hoang V, Anthony T, Gupta S, et al. Treatment of severe ankle and hindfoot deformity: technique using femoral head allograft for tibiotalocalcaneal fusion using a cup-and-cone reamer. Arthrosc Tech 2021;10(5):e1187–95.
16. Palmanovich E, Brin YS, Ben David D, et al. Use of a spinal cage for creating stable constructs in ankle and subtalar fusion. J Foot Ankle Surg 2015;54(2):254–7.
17. Preston NL, Wilson M, Hewitt EA. Salvage arthrodesis of a failed total ankle replacement using a custom 3D-printed cage implant: a case report and review of the literature. Proc Singapore Healthc 2018;27(4):277–81.
18. Hsu AR, Ellington JK. Patient-specific 3-dimensional printed titanium truss cage with tibiotalocalcaneal arthrodesis for salvage of persistent distal tibia nonunion. Foot Ankle Spec 2015;8:483–9.
19. Hamid KS, Parekh SG, Adams SB. Salvage of severe foot and ankle trauma with a 3D printed scaffold. Foot Ankle Int 2016;37:433–9.
20. Steele JR, Kadakia RJ, Cunningham DJ, et al. Comparison of 3D printed spherical implants versus femoral head allografts for tibiotalocalcaneal arthrodesis. J Foot Ankle Surg 2020;59(6):1167–70.
21. Dekker TJ, Steele JR, Federer AE, et al. Use of patient-specific 3D-Printed titanium implants for complex foot and ankle limb salvage, deformity correction, and arthrodesis procedures. Foot Ankle Int 2018;39(8):916–21.
22. Adams SB. Salvage arthrodesis for failed total ankle replacement. Foot Ankle Clin 2020;25(2):281–91.
23. Campana V, Milano G, Pagano E, et al. Bone substitutes in orthopedic surgery: from basic science to clinicalpractice. J Mater Sci Mater Med 2014;25:2445–61.

Updates on Total Ankle Arthroplasty

Jeffrey E. McAlister, DPM, Keegan A. Duelfer, DPM*

KEYWORDS

- Total ankle arthroplasty • Total ankle replacement • Patient-specific instrumentation
- TAR

KEY POINTS

- The third-generation and fourth-generation total ankle arthroplasty constructs exhibit high levels of long-term survivability with results similar to ankle arthrodesis procedures.
- Patient selection is paramount to implant survivability. Based on recent data there are very few absolute contraindications left for total ankle replacements; however, surgeons should constantly update their protocols for patient selection given the constant updating in the literature.
- The choices in total ankle replacement implants are plentiful. A number of these models are indicated for certain types of deformities, revision surgeries, and bone-sparing properties. Surgeon confidence in more than one model is ideal given these specializing features.

INTRODUCTION

The original total ankle implant system consisted of a long tibial stem with a polyethylene talar component, which necessitated a fusion of the subtalar joint.[1] The surgical technique was modeled after hip implants and would later be proven to poorly translate to total ankle implants in the long run. The official first-generation total ankle replacements (TARs) were the first to respect the native anatomy of the tibiotalar joint with their designs. This generation of implants consisted of a 2-component design with models varying from "constrained" to "non-constrained," depending on the polyethylene spacer without a separate independent bearing.[2,3] Unfortunately, this generation of TARs were plagued with high failure rates even in the short to mid-term results and were withdrawn from the market based on their high rates of subsidence, continued pain, and progressive deformity.

Despite these early fallbacks, innovation continued in this field and resulted in the next generation of implants being designed. These made use of metallic tibial and talar

Foot and Ankle Surgical Fellowship Program, Phoenix Foot and Ankle Institute, 7301 East 2nd Street Suite 206, Scottsdale, AZ 85251, USA
* Corresponding author.
E-mail address: duelfer1@gmail.com

Clin Podiatr Med Surg 40 (2023) 725–733
https://doi.org/10.1016/j.cpm.2023.05.013
0891-8422/23/© 2023 Elsevier Inc. All rights reserved.

components with an ultra-high molecular weight polyethylene. These generations from here on out could be subcategorized based on the number of components and device type. The 2-component systems are fixed bearing with the polyethylene spacer incorporated into the tibial component of the implant, whereas the 3-component systems are mobile bearing given their separate polyethylene spacer.

In conjunction with the adoption of the second and third generations came a newfound focus on reduction of bone resection and preservation of bone stock. The combination of newer implant design, surgeon education, and surgical technique based on evidence resulted in a dramatic increase in survivability of TARs. Complication rates have continued to decrease with this procedure, and for the first time, comparable complication rates and reoperation rates with ankle arthrodesis are being reported.[4–7]

The next stage in innovation has been recently introduced in the form of patient-specific instrumentation (PSI). These systems rely on CT scans that provide patient-specific and engineer-provided preoperative plan. This allows for the alignment and sizing of the metallic prosthetic component based on the patient's ankle joint landmarks or adjacent tibiotalar surface anatomy. With this information available in the preoperative phase, the surgeon can modify the plan based on their preferences or any additional cystic changes that may be near the intended TAR components. Upon final approval by the surgeon, the manufacturer creates a three-dimensional model of the patient's anatomy.

From these digital models a disposable physical cut guide is fabricated that allows the surgeon to avoid intramedullary or extramedullary guide set up because the patient-specific pinning and cutting guides do not need further referencing. Other potential benefits from this technique allow for less procedural complexity, less radiation, and less surgical time. Nonindustry sponsored research has noted low incidence of perfectly aligned PSI cut guides and only 77% accuracy within $\pm 5°$ from an axial rotational alignment.[8–12] To date comparison studies note that the PSI systems can get similar implant position and clinical outcomes to standard instrumentation but there is not strong enough evidence to date to evaluate PSI. It should also be noted that PSI has largely fallen out of favor in hip, knee, and shoulder arthroplasty given a reduction in accuracy.[13–19] These are factors that should be considered by the surgeon given the increased costs and health-care resources that are associated with PSI.

Patient Selection

The American Academy of Orthopaedic Surgeons have noted up to 14 factors that one should consider optimizing outcomes regarding surgical treatments of ankle arthritis. These factors include device type, patient age, patient weight, preoperative infection, fracture, surgical side, sex of patient, foot and ankle deformity, comorbidities, previous ankle surgery, presence of hindfoot arthritis, surgeon experience, and hospital surgical volume.

Gender

There is no influence of gender on total ankle survival.[20–22] Female gender was found to be a significant risk factor for wound healing problems but once corrected for confounding variables, it was no longer a predictor for disturbed wound healing.[23] Male gender is found to be a statistically significant risk factor for the occurrence of one or more complications within 30 days of surgery.[24]

Age

Younger age at implantation may affect the survivability of the implant in many ways. First, the TAR will need to function longer due to a higher life expectancy of the patient.

Additionally, younger patients tend to be more active, which has been proven to be associated with more wear of the prosthesis and polyethylene component. However, in a comparison study with the same implant patients aged younger than 50 years had a survival of 75% at 6.8 years and patients aged older than 50 years had a survival of 81% at 6 years with no statistically significant difference between the 2 groups.[25]

Activity level

Even though strong emphasis has been placed on the effect of activity level on the survivability of the implant research into this relationship is seldom performed. Now, there is no correlation between increased activity level and adverse effects with the Salto-Talaris, and Hintermann Prosthesis.[26,27] Despite the low number of research into this specific variable, guidelines have been developed that may be useful to discuss with the patient. These include continuation of aerobic or low impact sports and activities. Boot immobilized sports may be acceptable as long as patient has earlier experience with them. High impact, cutting, and jumping sports and activities are discouraged.[28]

Body mass index

Obesity was widely considered to be a contraindication for TAR. In the short-term postoperative phase, there are no statistical significant differences noted between complication rates and survivability among obese and nonobese patients with TAR.[29,30] In the moderate postoperative phase of 8 years, there are reports of 2.8 times higher chance of revision in obese patients compared with nonobese patients.[31] Most studies find that there is no correlation between BMI and results of TAR.

Smoking

Smoking again has been a contraindication of for TAR but there has only been one study that has investigated the relationship between smoking and TAR. In a retrospective review of 642 patients, there was a statistically significant increase in wound breakdown between the smokers versus nonsmokers.[32] Further research has been performed with an emphasis on less than 12 pack year smokers, which did not see a significant change in complication rates in smokers.

Comorbidities

To date, there is no literature that solidly supports the notion that diabetes should be considered a contraindication for TAR, apart from uncontrolled diabetes. No definitive statement could be made regarding neuropathy and vascular insufficiency due to lack of literature given their label as absolute contraindications.

Deformity

The importance of deformity correction either before or during TAR has been recognized quite some time.[33–36] Since the adoption of this guideline, the scientific evidence has strongly supported the notion that it is safe to assume that deformity is no longer a contraindication for TAR, if stepwise realignment procedures are followed accordingly.

Preoperative Planning

The preoperative planning process is an important part of the long-term success and survivability of the total ankle implant. This includes a full set of plain film radiographs including of the foot and ankle, hindfoot alignment, stress dorsiflexion, and stress plantarflexion. When performed correctly, these radiographs can help provide the foundation in determining the treatment of choice between fusion and replacement, as well as the true origin of the deformity. Along with a proper physical examination, this can help determine if the deformity is secondary to soft tissue or osseous rigidity. The determination for performing adjunctive deformity correction with a TAR versus staging deformity correction before implant placement can be chosen based on the amount of additional non–weight-bearing time each procedure is responsible for. To assist in optimizing range of motion of the implant, it is crucial to start physical therapy and weight-bearing as soon as possible, which is determined by the state of the anterior incision when solely a TAR is performed. The longer the non–weight-bearing and lack of range of motion on these patients with TAR, the more likely it is that the capsule will form adherences and that the other surrounding soft tissue will fibrose in a contracted position. Deformity correction through osseous procedures may add additional non–weight-bearing time in order to allow proper bone healing. If these additional adjunctive procedures are required to correct deformity, consideration for potential staging may be necessary. **Table 1** presents a broad protocol for staging, which has been used by the primary surgeon.[37]

CT scans are also vitally important to be performed in the preoperative stage to assess for cyst formation and bony abnormalities at the tibiotalar joint. Weight-bearing CT scans are applicable in this setting to determine ankle deformity in the stance of gait. Recent literature has explored the additional benefits of CT scans in the form of Hounsfield Unit measurements with their relation to bone mineral density. Studies specific in focus to the foot and ankle have determined bone attenuation of the distal tibia and talus on CT reveal significant correlation with bone mineral density (BMD) on all parts of a dual x-ray absorptiometry (DEXA) scan, and threshold HU values in the distal tibia and talus were defined for osteoporosis with the distal tibia at 122.5 and talus at 311.4.[38] Additionally, HU measurements have been related to risk of nonunion in ankle fractures and have also been used to define patients appropriate for prophylactic medial malleolar screw fixation during TAR procedures.[39,40]

Food and Drug Administration-Approved Systems

A brief description of the current TAR systems will be provided in the remaining article. An emphasis will be placed on the aspects of the system that are unique.

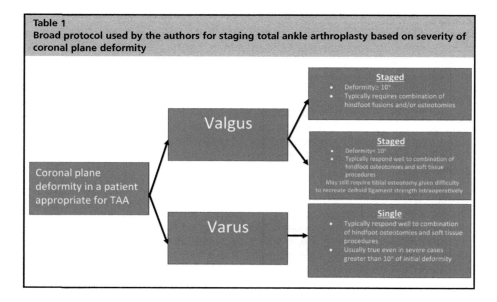

Table 1
Broad protocol used by the authors for staging total ankle arthroplasty based on severity of coronal plane deformity

Scandinavian Total Ankle Replacement

The second-generation scandinavian total ankle replacement (STAR) got Food and Drug Administration (FDA) approval in 2006, the first 3-component mobile-bearing implant in the United States, and for a long time, the only one available. Double-barrel tibial interface with a chamfer cuts talus and a central sagittal ridge that interacts with the polyethylene spacer. This system relies on an extramedullary tibial jig for establishing alignment of cuts into the tibia and talus. It remains one of the most well-studied systems and has demonstrated 80% to 90% survivorship at 10 years, 95.4% survivorship in one study at 12 years without cement use.[41–45] Sparse 15-year data show survivorship of 73%; however, this was determined from only 24 out of the 84 initial patients that were able to follow-up with the study.

Salto Talaris

Received FDA approval in 2006. Central keel for tibia fixation, which violates the anterior tiba for insertion. It mimics the anatomical articular surface of the talus by incorporating the curvature of the biconvex surfaces. It has a 5-year survivability of 95.8%. The Salto Talaris XT Revision ankle prosthesis is a fixed bearing system with an option for a central keel to reduce bone loss, and the ultra-high molecular weight polyethylene (UHMWPE) spacer has more options to assist in these revision cases.

Inbone II

Gained FDA approval 2010 and was largely evolved from the same concepts as the Inbone I model. This is a 2-component fixed bearing system with an intramedullary tibial stem of variable length. This system has been reported to have a 98% survivorship at 5 years.[46] There is no chamfer option with this device and contains additional talar dome "pegs" to provide additional fixation in the talus and a sulcus talar design.

Infinity

A fourth-generation system. This 2-component fixed bearing device in compatible with the Inbone II and Invision systems by design. This design retained the same talar sulcus as the Inbone II but unlike this older system does not contain the intramedullary stems or large external jig. There is a PSI option for this system known as the Prophecy. Short-term survivability for this system at 1.8 years has been shown in recent literature to be 98.2%.[47]

Invision

Developed as a purely revision system for the Inbone II and Infinity systems. Consists of a 2-component fixed system with multiple areas of built-in variability. The tibial component consists of an intramedullary tibial stem of variable length, whereas the polyethylene spacer comes in sizes ranging from 2 to 6 mm. Additionally, the talar plate also has 2 thickness options for the restoration of joint height as well as a broadened anterior lip to provide additional purchase into the talar neck.

Zimmer trabecular metal total ankle replacement

Cleared by the FDA 2012. Third-generation 2-component replacement with a transfibular approach. It is the only laterally based total ankle system in use in the United States. This technique avoids the typical anterior-based incision in order to prevent wound healing issues. External jig utilized. Instead of a standard flat tibial cut, this tibial component follows the natural anterior to posterior curve of the distal articular surface given this unique lateral approach technique. The talar component has a medial to laterally based radius of curvature to allow axial motion. It uses a highly cross-linked polyethylene (HXPLE) spacer that may have decreased wear and less debris.

Recent literature has shown that at an average of 24 months, the survivability is at 93% for this system.[48]

Vantage
This system received FDA approval in 2016. It offers detailed tibial and talar anatomically shaped implants with a unique cage peg to allow for bony ingrowth. Has both 2-component and 3-component designs.

Cadence
This system received FDA approval in 2016. It is a fourth-generation 2-component fixed bearing system. Currently, the 2-year survivorship is at 93.7%.[49] There are chamfer and flat cut talus options with plans in the near future to allow for a PSI system. There is a fibular groove in the tibial component and allows for posterior and anterior correction of the implant. Uses an HXPLE spacer for greater durability.

Hintermann
The Hintermann Series H2 received FDA approval in 2017, whereas the Hintermann Series H3 received approval in 2019. The H2 is a semiconstrained 2-component implant while the H3 is a nonconstrained mobile bearing 3-component system. These both contain a UHMWPE spacer and allow for chamfer and flat cut talus types.

Apex 3D
Cleared by the FDA in 2020. Low-profile tibial component with 2 pegs placed more posteriorly from midline to engage peak bone density of the tibia. The polyethylene spacer is infused with Vitamin E with the purposes of reducing oxidation, debris, and osteolysis, and this spacer can disengage from the tibial component for potential exchange. The talar component comes with a flat cut and chamfered guide. There are 3 options for cut guides with a traditional extramedullary that spans the length of the tibia, an abbreviated cut guide that is pinned solely along the tibiotalar joint and a PSI system.

Kinos
Cleared by the FDA in 2020. First to employ a saddle-shaped articular surface to decrease implant wear and to allow adequate inversion/eversion, and internal/external rotation as the physiologic ankle does. The tibial and talar components come available with a left and right model due to the saddle type surface that allows for triplanar motion.

CLINICS CARE POINTS

- Although very few absolute contraindication exist in the implantation of a TAR, it is important to consider the following patient characteristics: gender, age, activity level, BMI, smoking, and comorbidities.

- Performing a complete workup of the patient in the preoperative setting is paramount to long-term total ankle arthroplasty success. Certain physical examination findings and imaging modalities are important to evaluate deformity and its level, cystic changes to either the tibia or talus and bone mineral assessment.

- An intimate understanding of the different total ankle systems is necessary. The most important aspect of these designs to understand include the specific specializations and indications that are assigned to certain models because this will help in selecting the most appropriate implant for any given patient.

DISCLOSURE

The authors have nothing to disclose.

REFERENCES

1. Lord G, Marotte JH. Total ankle prosthesis. Technic and 1st results. Apropos of 12 cases. Rev Chir Orthop Reparatrice Appar Mot 1973;59(2):139–51.
2. Gougoulias NE, Khanna A, Maffulli N. History and evolution in total ankle arthroplasty. Br Med Bull 2009;89:111–51.
3. Gougoulias N, Maffulli N. History of total ankle replacement. Clin Podiatr Med Surg 2013;30(1):1–20.
4. Kim J, Rajan L, Bitar R. Early Radiographic and Clinical Outcomes of a Novel, Fixed- Bearing Fouth- Generation Total Ankle Replacement System. Foot and Ankle International 2022;43(11):1424–33.
5. Kim HJ, Suh DH, Yang JH, et al. Total ankle arthroplasty versus ankle arthrodesis for the treatment of end-stage ankle arthritis: a meta- analysis of comparative studies. Int Orthop 2017;41(1):101–9.
6. Cody EA, Scott DJ, Easley ME. Total ankle arthroplasty: a critical analysis review. JBJS Rev 2018;6(8):e8.
7. Fanelli D, Mercurio M, Castioni D, et al. End-stage ankle osteoarthritis: arthroplasty offers better quality of life than arthrodesis with similar complication and re-operation rates-an updated meta-analysis of comparative studies. Int Orthop 2021;45(9):2177–91.
8. Escudero MI, Symes M, Bemenderfer TB, et al. Does patient-specific instrumentation have a higher rate of early osteolysis than standard referencing techniques in total ankle arthroplasty? A radiographic analysis. Foot Ankle Spec 2020;13: 32–42.
9. Najefi A-A, Goldberg A. The role of axial rotation in total ankle replacement. Foot Ankle Orthop 2018. https://doi.org/10.1177/2F2473011418S00090.
10. Gagne OJ, Veljkovic A, Townshend D, et al. Intraoperative assessment of the axial rotational positioning of a modern ankle arthroplasty tibial component using preoperative patient-specific instrumentation guidance. Foot Ankle Int 2019;40: 1160–5.
11. Hintermann B, Susdorf R, Krähenbühl N, et al. Axial rotational alignment of mobile-bearing total ankle arthroplasty. Foot Ankle Int 2020;41:521–8.
12. Ciudo DJ, Baker EA, Fortin PT. Tibial torsion may predict morphology of the talus. Foot Ankle Orthop 2020. https://doi.org/10.1177/2F2473011420S00171.
13. Henckel J, Holme T, Warwick R, et al. 3D-printed patient-specific guides for hip arthroplasty. J Am Acad Orthop Surg 2018;26:e342–8.
14. Thienpont E, Schwab PE, Fennema P. A systematic review and meta-anlalysis of patient-specific instrumentation for improving alignment of the components in total knee replacement. Bone Joint Lett J 2014;96-B:1052–61.
15. Kosse N, Heesterbeek PJC, Schimmel JJP, et al. Stability and alignment do not improve by using patient-specific instrumentation in total knee arthroplasty: a randomized controlled trial. Knee Surg Sports Traumatol Arthrosc 2018;26:1792–9.
16. Abane L, Zaoui A, Anract P, et al. Can a single-use and patient-specific instrumentation be reliably used in primary total knee arthroplasty? A multicenter controlled study. J Arthroplasty 2018;33:2111–8.
17. Kizaki K, Shanmugaraj A, Yamashita F. Total knee arthroplasty using patient-specific instrumentation for osteoarthritis of the knee: a meta-analysis. BMC BMC MusculoskelDisord 2019;20:561.

18. Lau SC, Keith PPA. Patient-specific instrumentation for total shoulder arthroplasty: not as accurate as it would seem. J Shoulder Elbow Surg 2018;2:90–5.
19. Cabarcas BC, Cvetanovich GL, Gowd AK, et al. Accuracy of patient-specific instrumentation in shoulder arthroplasty: a systematic review and meta-analysis. JSES Open Access 2019;3:117–29.
20. Henricson A, Skoog A, Carlsson A. The Swedish ankle arthroplasty register: an analysis of 531 arthroplasties between 1993 and 2005. Acta Orthop 2007; 78(5):569–74.
21. Skyttä ET, Koivu H, Eskelinen A, et al. Total ankle replacement: a population-based study of 515 cases from the Finnish Arthroplasty Register. Acta Orthop 2010;81(1):114–8.
22. Hosman AH, Mason RB, Hobbs T, et al. A New Zealand national joint registry review of 202 total ankle replacements followed for up to 6 years. Acta Orthop 2007;78(5):584–91.
23. Raikin SM, Kane J, Ciminiello ME. Risk factors for incision-healing complications following total ankle arthroplasty. J Bone Joint Surg Am 2010;92(12):2150–5.
24. Zhou H, Yakavonis M, Shaw JJ, et al. In-patient trends and complications after total ankle arthroplasty in the United States. Orthopedics 2016;39(1):e74–9.
25. Kofoed H, Lundberg-Jensen A. Ankle arthroplasty in patients younger and older than 50 years: a prospective series with long-term follow-up. Foot Ankle Int 1999; 20(8):501–6.
26. Naal FD, Impellizzeri FM, Loibl M, et al. Habitual physical activity and sports participation after total ankle arthroplasty. Am J Sports Med 2009;37(1):95–102.
27. Bonnin MP, Laurent JR, Casillas M. Ankle function and sports activity after total ankle arthroplasty. Foot Ankle Int 2009;30(10):933–44.
28. Macaulay AA, VanValkenburg SM, DiGiovanni CW. Sport and activity restrictions following total ankle replacement: a survey of orthopaedic foot and ankle specialists. Foot Ankle Surg 2015;21(4):260–5.
29. Barg A, Knupp M, Anderson AE, et al. Total ankle replacement in obese patients: component stability, weight change, and functional outcome in 118 consecutive patients. Foot Ankle Int 2011;32(10):925–32.
30. Bouchard M, Amin A, Pinsker E, et al. The impact of obesity on the outcome of total ankle replacement. J Bone Joint Surg Am 2015;97(11):904–10.
31. Schipper ON, Denduluri SK, Zhou Y, et al. Effect of obesity on total ankle arthroplasty outcomes. Foot Ankle Int 2016;37(1):1–7.
32. Lampley A, Gross CE, Green CL, et al. Association of cigarette use and complication rates and outcomes following total ankle arthroplasty. Foot Ankle Int 2016; 37(10):1052–9.
33. Greisberg J, Hansen ST Jr. Ankle replacement: management of associated deformities. Foot Ankle Clin 2002;7(4):721–36, vi.
34. Stamatis ED, Myerson MS. How to avoid specific complications of total ankle replacement. Foot Ankle Clin 2002;7(4):765–89.
35. Wood PL, Sutton C, Mishra V, et al. A randomised, controlled trial of two mobile-bearing total ankle replacements. J Bone Joint Surg Br 2009;91(1):69–74.
36. de Asla RJ, Ellis S, Overley B, et al. Total ankle arthroplasty in the setting of valgus deformity. Foot Ankle Spec 2014;7(5):398–402.
37. Duelfer K, McAlister J. Appropriate staging techniques in total ankle reconstruction. Foot Ankle Surg: Techniques, Reports, and Cases 2023;3(1):10–6.
38. Lee SY, Kwon SS, Kim HS, et al. Reliability and validity of lower extremity computed tomography as a screening tool for osteoporosis. Osteoporos Int 2015;26:1387–94.

39. Cody EA, Lachman JR, Gausden EB. Lower bone density on preoperative computed tomography predicts periprosthetic fracture risk in total ankle arthroplasty. Foot Ankle Int 2018;40:1–8.
40. Stowers JM, Black AT, Kavanagh AM, et al. Predicting nonunions in ankle fractures using quantitative tibial hounsfield samples from preoperative computed tomography: a multicenter matched case control study. J Foot Ankle Surg 2021. https://doi.org/10.1053/j.jfas.2021.10.007. S1067-2516(21)00395-1.
41. Saltzman CL, Mann RA, Ahrens JE, et al. Prospective controlled trial of STAR total ankle replacement versus ankle fusion: initial results. Foot Ankle Int 2009;30(7): 579–96.
42. Kofoed H. Scandinavian total ankle replacement (STAR). Clin Orthop Relat Res 2004;424:73–9.
43. Mann JA, Mann RA, Horton E. STAR ankle: long-term results. Foot Ankle Int 2011; 32(5):S473–84.
44. Nunley JA, Caputo AM, Easley ME, et al. Intermediate to long-term outcomes of the STAR Total Ankle Replacement: the patient perspective. J Bone Joint Surg Am 2012;94(1):43–8.
45. Wood PL, Prem H, Sutton C. Total ankle replacement: medium-term results in 200 Scandinavian total ankle replacements. J Bone Joint Surg Br 2008;90(5):605–9.
46. Gagne O, Day J, Kim J. Midterm survivorship of the inbone II total ankle arthroplasty. FAI 2021;43(5):628–36.
47. Rushing CJ, Kibbler K, Hyer CF, et al. The INFINITY total ankle prosthesis: outcomes at short term follow up. Foot Ankle Spec 2022;15(2):119–26.
48. Barg A, Bettin C, Burstein AH, et al. Early clinical and radiographic outcomes of trabecular metal total ankle replacement using a transfibular approach. J Bone Joint Surg Am 2018;100(6):505–15.
49. Kim J, Rajan L, Bitar R, et al. Early radiographic and clinical outcomes of a novel, fixed-bearing fourth-generation total ankle replacement system. FAI 2022;43(11): 1424–33.

Management of Talar Avascular Necrosis with Total Talus

James M. Cottom, DPM, FACFAS[a],*, Jay S. Badell, DPM, AACFAS[a],
Joseph R. Wolf, DPM, AACFAS[a]

KEYWORDS

- Total talus • Avascular necrosis • 3D printing • Ankle arthritis • Talus replacement

KEY POINTS

- Avascular necrosis of the talus leaves the surgeon with limited treatment options for a functional foot and ankle.
- The advent of patient-specific 3D printed implants provides an avenue for the patient to maintain joint range of motion and function of the ankle.
- Several techniques are available to remove the native talus; however, care should be taken to protect the surrounding soft tissue and bony structures to ensure maximum stability of the newly implanted custom talus.
- Evidence is limited with regard to total talus due to the novelty of the technology; however, it provides a viable option in cases of avascular necrosis of the talus.

BACKGROUND

Avascular necrosis (AVN) can be a devastating condition regardless of location throughout the body. AVN of the talus can be an exceptionally challenging entity to treat due to the repetitive loading of the foot and ankle during daily activity. Talar AVN can have several etiologies, but is most commonly seen following trauma that disrupts the tenuous blood supply to the bone.[1–3] Talar neck and body fractures in particular are responsible for a large number of cases of talar AVN, with adjacent joint dislocations increasing the risk for osteonecrosis.[2,4,5] High dose systemic steroids, bone tumors, previous failed total ankle arthroplasty have also shown to be a causative factor leading to AVN of the talus.[3,5,6]

The patient typically presents with diffuse ankle pain which is increased with ambulation, and progressive in nature. Imaging studies are critical for evaluation, and usually begin with standard radiographs. The surgeon may be able to detect old fractures

[a] Florida Orthopedic Foot & Ankle Center, 5741 Bee Ridge Road, Suite 490, Sarasota, FL 34233, USA
* Corresponding author. 5741 Bee Ridge Road, #490, Sarasota, FL 34243.
E-mail address: jamescottom300@gmail.com

Clin Podiatr Med Surg 40 (2023) 735–747
https://doi.org/10.1016/j.cpm.2023.05.014
0891-8422/23/© 2023 Elsevier Inc. All rights reserved.
podiatric.theclinics.com

or implanted hardware from previous fracture repair. Sclerotic changes are usually seen within the talus on plain radiographs depending on the time from injury. MRI (**Fig. 1**) and/or CT (**Fig. 2**) are then regularly ordered for further evaluation of bony integrity and treatment planning.[1] The Ficat classification (**Table 1**) can be of use when evaluating imaging to guide treatment.[5,6]

Conservative treatment consists of protected weight bearing or immobilization of the affected limb, bracing. Shock wave therapy has shown some improvement in symptoms in cases of AVN of the femoral head,[7] however data is limited with regard to the talus. Previous studies have shown some effectiveness of treatment with complete non-weight bearing; however, the duration of immobilization needed to see improvement was minimum three months.[5] Immobilization for such an extended period of time can have other deleterious effects on the body and patient well-being. Newer technology and regenerative medicine techniques can also be utilized such as PRP, BMA, or amniotic injections.[3,5] Conservative therapy can be effective for a period of time in the early stages of AVN prior to bony collapse, but patients usually require some form of surgical treatment due to the progressive nature of arthritis and pain.[5]

Joint preserving procedures may be attempted in cases where bony integrity is still maintained. These include bone grafting or core decompression.[5,8] Joint destructive procedures include talectomy with blair fusion of the tibia directly to the calcaneus, or the traditional tibiotalocalcaneal arthrodesis using structural bone allograft or custom printed cages. These methods have been shown to lead to an increase of adjacent joint arthritis in patients with pre-existing, asymptomatic arthritis.[9]

Ultimately a lengthy discussion is performed with the patient regarding whichever treatment options are planned including risks and benefits of each treatment. The authors prefer to maintain joint motion whenever feasible, which is where the advent of custom-printed total talus has provided a legitimate alternative to joint destructive surgery. Talus replacements are currently in the third generation of their existence with most common compositions of cobalt chrome or aluminum.[10] Several other metal alloys have also been reported in the literature.

CT scans of the ipsilateral and contralateral talus are used to create a custom, patient-specific recreation for accurate anatomic fit. Engineers with the industry partner of choice receive the scans and typically have a conference with the surgeon within 1-2 weeks. This includes the initial surgical plan, and surgeon can provide feedback and make any necessary changes they see fit at this time. Production team then creates a computer-generated representation of the patient's talus, along with a surgical guide (**Fig. 3**). This includes such details as visuals of repositioned anatomy post native talus resection, trial sizers, and final implant using nominal as well as additional sizes (**Figs. 4** and **5**). Once the surgeon and engineer agree on the implant and plan, the talus is custom printed. This process takes approximately 4-6 weeks from

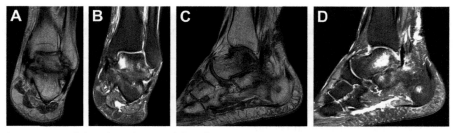

Fig. 1. Coronal (*A, B*) and sagittal (*C, D*) MRI views in patient with large cystic changes within the body of the talus after fracture which was treated conservatively.

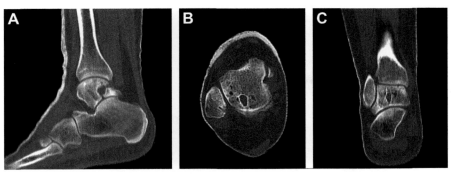

Fig. 2. Sagittal (*A*), axial (*B*), and coronal (*C*) CT views in patient with large cystic changes within posterior body of talus.

proposal to TTR surgery, depending on industry partner. The end goal of talus replacement surgery is return to activities of daily living with decreased pain and without the use of ambulatory aids.

Surgical Techniques

In cases with a previous wound infection, a staged approach may be necessary to limit complications. The authors recommend a first-stage resection of talus, bone biopsy, wound debridement, and closure with the placement of antibiotic cement spacer (**Fig. 6**). Antibiotic cement spacer is left in place for 6 weeks with simultaneous administration of intravenous antibiotics. At this point, if infection is ruled out, the surgeon may proceed with the next steps of care.

- Incisional approach for custom total talus involves a standard anterior ankle incision with dissection through the superior extensor retinaculum. Dissection is carried down to the level of the tibialis anterior and extensor hallucis longus tendons. Anterior compartment tendons are maintained within their sheath whenever possible. Dissection is carried down just medial to the neurovascular structures which typically lie deep to the extensor hallucis longus tendon. The neurovascular structures are carefully maintained within their fatty adipose tissue. An anterior capsulotomy is performed with the resection of any redundant anterior capsule. Deep retraction is utilized with Gelpi or Weitlaner retractors with care to avoid the superficial soft tissues. There is often significant scar tissue present which needs to be resected in order to increase motion about the ankle.

Table 1 Ficat classification for stages of talar osteonecrosis using radiographic and MRI findings		
Ficat classification for the stage of talar osteonecrosis		
Factor	Radiographic Findings	MRI Findings
Stage 1	Normal	Mild Marrow Edema
Stage 2	Sclerosis and/or Cystic Lesions	More defined Osteonecrosis
Stage 3	Crescent Sign, Subchondral Collapse of Talar Dome	Diffuse Edema Surround Osteonecrosis
Stage 4	Arthritis of Tibiotalar Joint, Loss of Joint Space, Osteophytes	Cartilage Loss/Thinning, Marrow Edema at Tibial Plafond

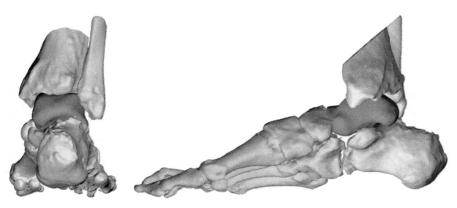

Proposed medium implant represents 95% the volume of the contralateral talus.

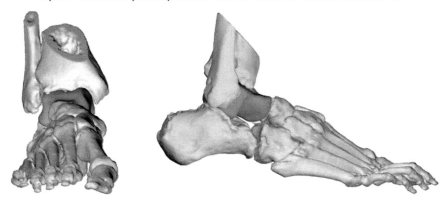

Proposed medium implant represents 95% the volume of the contralateral talus.

Fig. 3. Pre-Operative surgical guide displaying the positioning of the nominal talus implant.

- Multiple techniques have been described to resect the talus. One can utilize a combination of an osteotome and rongeur to excise and piecemeal the talus. Additionally, a meniscotome and Cobb elevator can be utilized to circumferentially release capsular attachments, especially posterior, followed by removal of the talus with a Steinmann or Schanz pin (**Fig. 7**). Alternate technique to remove the native talus is to utilize a sagittal saw to osteotomize the talus into thirds, orienting the saw to create an anteriorly based wedge. One can then easily remove the central wedge which has no soft tissue attachment, thus creating more room and visualization to carefully remove the remaining bone.
- An important step of the procedure is to release the posterior ankle joint capsule with a cautery or surgical blade to allow greater motion. The authors also recommend being very conscientious about leaving the deep deltoid attachment to the calcaneus intact and the calcaneofibular ligament laterally. It is also recommended to resect any osteophytes or hypertrophic bone on the dorsal navicular, tibia, and fibula.
- After removal of the diseased talus, the talar trial implants can then be inserted. Several trial sizers are usually available to obtain optimal fit. This typically includes a nominal trial, and trials of 5% larger and 5% smaller than nominal.

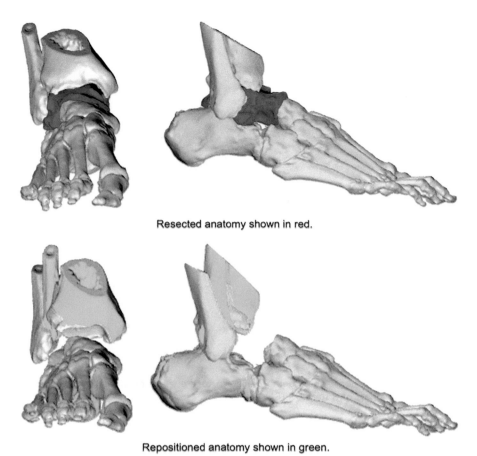

Resected anatomy shown in red.

Repositioned anatomy shown in green.

Fig. 4. Example of surgical guide provided by engineers in pre-operative planning phase. Area in red displays the bone that is to be removed and area in green displays the ability to restore anatomy after removal of the diseased talus.

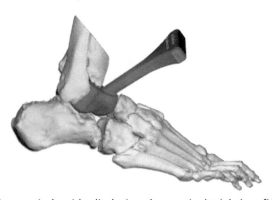

Fig. 5. Pre-operative surgical guide displaying the nominal trial sizer fit within the ankle mortise.

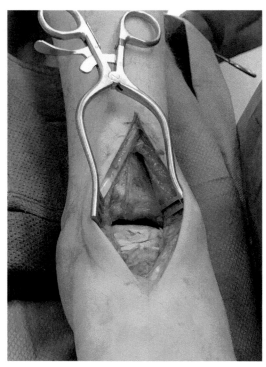

Fig. 6. Antibiotic cement spacer being placed in to the space previously occupied by the native talus as a part of a staged TTR.

This allows for any intraoperative changes that may need to be performed or changes that are seen intraoperatively (**Fig. 8**). The authors have found the orientation of the trial sizer handle can interfere with the proper assessment of ankle joint range of motion and stability. In this case, the handle can be removed using a sagittal saw. The nominal size is most commonly chosen and utilized (**Figs. 9** and **10**).

- Presurgical planning process involves the customization of suture hole placement for any soft tissue attachments per surgeon's discretion and optional interfaces for screw heads if a subtalar/talonavicular joint arthrodesis is to be performed concomitantly (**Fig. 11**). If lateral ankle ligament repair is chosen to be performed through the implant, the appropriate suture interface sites are utilized on the lateral aspect of the newly implanted talus at this time (**Fig. 12**). The

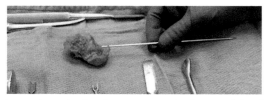

Fig. 7. Entirety of the native talus has been removed using careful soft tissue release and utilization of a Schanz pin.

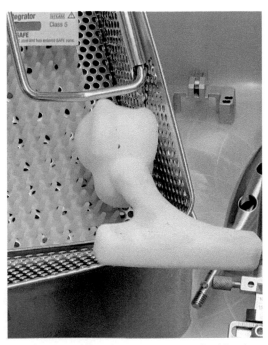

Fig. 8. Nominal talus trial sizer used to determine proper final implant size.

authors recommend threading suture through the interface on the talus prior to final implantation. Attempting to perform this step after implantation can be diffi-cult due to limited space.

- The authors prefer to reinforce the lateral ankle ligaments after the custom talus has been implanted utilizing an alternate method. This is done by performing an Evans peroneal rerouting. A small additional incision is made posterior to the fib-ula above the level of the ankle. The peroneal retinaculum is incised and the per-oneus brevis tendon is isolated. The tendon is then carefully split, whipstitched, and rerouted distally to the level of the ankle using a hemostat or suture passer. The surgeon can then either opt to perform the tendon transfer and lateral ankle ligament repair through the anterior ankle incision or a small accessory incision at the level of the lateral malleolus. The authors rationale for non-anatomic type lateral ankle ligament repair is creating a native tissue to tissue repair, rather than solely relying on soft tissue to metal implant adherence.

- At this time the operative site is thoroughly irrigated. Final C-arm images are taken and a posterior muscle group lengthening is performed at this time if needed. The incision is closed in layers including the anterior capsule, extensor retinaculum, subcutaneous tissue, and skin. A Robert Jones cotton dressing is then applied with appropriate compression.

- There are currently no dedicated guidelines for the postoperative management of talus replacement. Patients are seen back in the clinic in approximately 2 weeks where the splint is changed. The incision and soft tissues are monitored very carefully and a tall weightbearing CAM walker boot is initiated once the incision is healed. This is usually four to six weeks post-operatively. Physical therapy is then started as soon as the incision is healed. The patient may transition out of

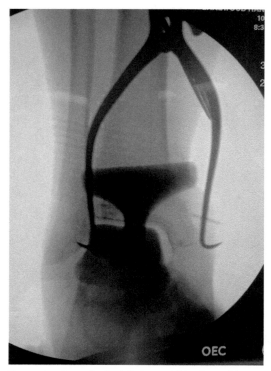

Fig. 9. Ankle AP radiograph of nominal trial sizer within the ankle mortise.

the cam walker boot after completing 4-6 sessions of physical therapy and is transitioned into a functional lace up brace with an athletic shoe. Radiographs are taken at 2 weeks, 6 weeks, 3 months, 6 months, and 1 year (**Figs. 13** and **14**). If adjunct procedures are performed, postoperative weightbearing protocol is modified accordingly.

DISCUSSION

Treatment options for talar AVN have traditionally been geared toward arthrodesis procedures. This usually involves a tibiotalocalcaneal fusion, which have had poor union rates compared to other arthrodesis procedures in the foot and ankle. With the non-union rate of TTC fusion being as high as 40%,[9,11] alternative options were heavily sought after in patients with end stage AVN of the talus. The potential of a treatment option that avoids fusion about the talus while maintaining ankle range of motion is attractive to both patients and surgeons.

3D printed prostheses have just recently entered the surgical and medical arena, but have already shown great promise to treat a wide range of conditions.[10] Originally, 3D printing was used to demonstrate anatomy and help with pre-surgical planning. In the present day, this technology has allowed for the creation of patient-specific implants to replace diseased areas of the body. This is exceptionally useful in the field of orthopedic surgery. As technology continues to become more advanced, the usefulness to medical professionals and surgeons in particular will similarly increase.

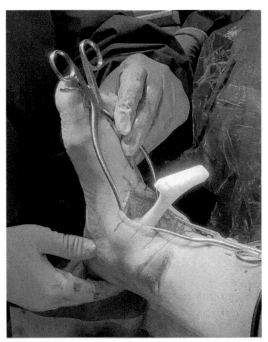

Fig. 10. Nominal trial sizer has been inserted into ankle mortise, surgeon is performing the range of motion about the ankle joint and assessing stability.

More specifically, 3D printed custom total talus are currently in the 3rd generation of implants, and could still be considered in its infancy.[10] More recent studies have begun to show promise with the technology, with patient outcomes and pain drastically improving post-operatively. Evidence is being gathered more quickly in favor of TTR with increased numbers of surgical cases taking place worldwide.

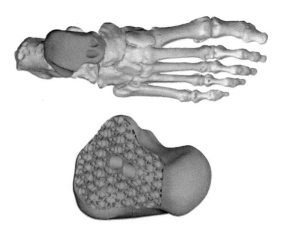

Fig. 11. Options exist to further customize the printed talus. This example shows the addition of subtalar joint screw holes, and porous design of the inferior talus for arthrodesis.

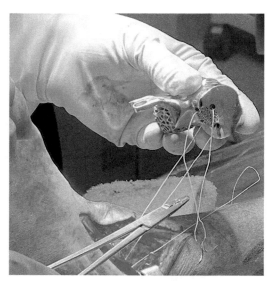

Fig. 12. Custom Interface within the talus has been created to allow the suture to be passed for lateral ankle ligament reconstruction.

Scott and colleagues[11] retrospectively reviewed 15 patients who underwent total talus replacement over a two-year period. Patient outcomes reviewed included radiographic alignment, FAOS scores, VAS score, and ankle range of motion with an average follow up time of 12.8 months. They found statistically significant decrease of VAS (7.0 to 3.6), and improved FAOS scores. Radiographic alignment did not change from pre-op to post-op. There was a trend toward increased subtalar and ankle joint range of motion, however this was not statistically significant. They concluded that total talus replacement showed good short-term outcomes with improved functional patient outcome scores and improvement in pain. They also showed 100% survivorship of the implant at final follow-up. The authors did endorse the limitation of small sample size; however, this is due in large part to the novelty of the procedure.

Kadakia and colleagues[3] also retrospectively reviewed 27 patients undergoing TTR over a three-year period. They reviewed FAOS scores, VAS scores, ankle range of motion, as well as postoperative complications for an average follow-up time of

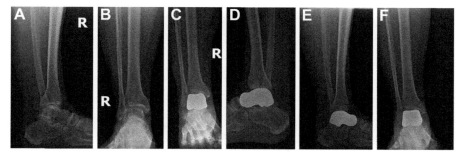

Fig. 13. Ankle AP and lateral pre-operative radiographs of patient with talar AVN secondary to cystic changes within the body of the talus (*A, B*). Ankle AP and lateral 2-week postoperative radiographs (*C, D*). Ankle AP and lateral 6-month post-operative radiographs (*E, F*).

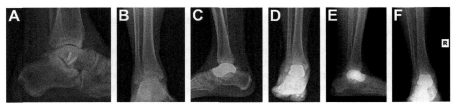

Fig. 14. Ankle AP and lateral pre-operative radiographs of patient with post-traumatic talar AVN due to previous talar body fracture and ORIF (A, B). Ankle AP and lateral 2-week post-operative radiographs (C, D). Ankle AP and lateral 6-month post-operative radiographs (E, F).

22.2 months. This study found statistically significant changes including an improvement of VAS (7.1 to 3.9) as well as increased FAOS scores in pain, symptoms, quality of life, and activities of daily living. Ankle range of motion was unchanged when compared to pre-operative measurements. They did have three complications requiring reoperation which included a superficial peroneal neuroma which required surgical excision, a superficial infection which required irrigation and debridement and foot reconstruction for residual deformity. This patient elected to undergo below knee amputation due to persistent pain. The final complication was the collapse of the distal tibia due to AVN and was converted to tibiotalocalcaneal arthrodesis. The authors concluded that TTR is a viable unique surgical option to maintain motion in patients with talar AVN.

Tracey and colleagues[12] performed a unique study retrospectively analyzing radiographic alignment measurements of 14 patients who underwent TTR over a two-year period. The study used plain radiographs to measure pre-operative and post-operative native talar dimensions, custom implanted talar dimensions, and corresponding measurements about the ankle, rearfoot, and forefoot. Measurements included tibiotalar alignment, talar declination, Boehler's angle, and Meary's angle. The authors found that talar arc, length, and width were not significantly changed. However, they did find that post-operative talar height was significantly increased. Only talar tilt was found to be significantly changed in radiographic measurements. The authors attribute this to asymmetric collapse of the native talus. They ultimately concluded that TTR maintains normal anatomy and alignment while restoring talar height.

SUMMARY

The ability to accurately match the patient's native anatomy, maintain motion, and customize care to meet every patient's specific needs is a valuable tool when discussing treatment options in the case of talar AVN. The current applications for TTR are becoming more versatile, with options to customize the talus for adjacent joint fusions and ligament repairs. TTR has also been utilized in events of talar AVN compounded by adjacent tibial plafond arthritis. The option exists to combine a total talus replacement with tibial prosthesis, also known as total ankle total talus replacement (TATTR).[13] TTR is being utilized more commonly by todays surgeons, and has shown promise as a viable long-term solution in cases of avascular necrosis of the talus.

CLINICS CARE POINTS

- Not all patients are appropriate for TTR. Careful selection and attempt at conservative and alternate surgical therapies must be performed. If decision is made to proceed with TTR,

MRI, and CT are essential in surgical planning and assessment of bony and soft tissue structures about the ankle joint.

- Excision of the diseased native talus can be performed using several different techniques. Cobb or meniscotome can be used to free the talus from all soft tissue attachments, and Schanz pin can be inserted to remove the talus in its entirety. The talus can be removed piecemeal using rongeur and osteotome. A sagittal saw can also be used to divide the talus into thirds.

- Regardless of techniques used to remove the native talus, it is critical in the authors opinion to leave the deltoid ligament and calcaneofibular ligament fully intact to maintain stability about the ankle joint.

- The authors prefer to perform a release of the posterior ankle capsule to allow for great sagittal plane motion about the ankle joint. Large amounts of scar tissue and hypertrophic bone can be present in patients with longstanding arthritis, and failure to remove the redundant tissue could limit ankle joint motion during the post-operative period.

- Length and orientation of the trial sizer handles may hinder the surgeon's ability to properly assess the trial talus. In this case, the authors recommend removing the handle using a sagittal saw to properly assess ankle range of motion and stability.

- Reinforcement of the lateral ankle ligaments must be assessed with every TTR. Pre-operative planning with industry engineers includes options for suture anchor placement within the custom implant. If interface within the talus is chosen, the surgeon should thread the suture prior to final implantation. The authors prefer to utilize the Evans peroneal rerouting to reinforce the lateral ankle ligaments so as not to solely rely on the adherence of soft tissues to a metal implant.

- Anterior ankle incision wound closure is performed in layers in the same manner as the traditional anterior approach for total ankle replacement or fusion. Meticulous extensor retinaculum closure is exceptionally important due to close apposition to the tendinous and neurovascular structures that lie just deep to this layer. Proper post-operative monitoring of incisions and edema are critical, as wound dehiscence and deep infection can have potentially disastrous results such as implant removal, prolonged IV antibiotics, and potentially leg amputation.

- Patients are typically placed into a splint post-operatively and quickly transitioned into a weightbearing tall walking boot once the incision is healed and the soft tissue envelope allows. Early range of motion and progression to weight bearing is encouraged to prevent the formation of scar tissue and ankle contracture. Physical therapy is also encouraged once incisions have healed to support the maintenance of range of motion.

- Talar AVN can be a difficult pathology to treat.

- Total Talus replacements may provide to be a good option, but mid-term and long-term data is lacking.

DISCLOSURES

None.

REFERENCES

1. Couturier S, Gold G. Imaging features of avascular necrosis of the foot and ankle. Foot Ankle Clin 2019;24(1):17–33.
2. Dodd A, Lefaivre KA. Outcomes of talar neck fractures: a systematic review and meta-analysis. J Orthop Trauma 2015;29(5):210–5.
3. Kadakia RJ, Akoh CC, Chen J, et al. 3D printed total talus replacement for avascular necrosis of the talus. Foot Ankle Int 2020;41(12):1529–36.

4. Chiodo CP, Herbst SA. Osteonecrosis of the talus. Foot Ankle Clin 2004 Dec;9(4): 745–55, vi.

5. Parekh SG, Kadakia RJ. Avascular necrosis of the talus. J Am Acad Orthop Surg 2021;29(6):e267–78.

6. Haskell A. Natural history of avascular necrosis in the talus: when to operate. Foot Ankle Clin 2019;24(1):35–45.

7. Vulpiani MC, Vetrano M, Trischitta D, et al. Extracorporeal shock wave therapy in early osteonecrosis of the femoral head: prospective clinical study with long-term follow-up. Arch Orthop Trauma Surg 2012;132(4):499–508.

8. Gross CE, Haughom B, Chahal J, et al. Treatments for avascular necrosis of the talus: a systematic review. Foot Ankle Spec 2014;7(5):387–97.

9. Ling JS, Smyth NA, Fraser EJ, et al. Investigating the relationship between ankle arthrodesis and adjacent-joint arthritis in the hindfoot: a systematic review. J Bone Joint Surg Am 2015;97(6):513–20.

10. Kadakia RJ, Wixted CM, Allen NB, et al. Clinical applications of custom 3D printed implants in complex lower extremity reconstruction. 3D Print Med. 2020;6(1):29.

11. Scott DJ, Steele J, Fletcher A, et al. Early outcomes of 3D printed total talus arthroplasty. Foot Ankle Spec 2020;13(5):372–7.

12. Tracey J, Arora D, Gross CE, et al. Custom 3D-printed total talar prostheses restore normal joint anatomy throughout the hindfoot. Foot Ankle Spec 2019; 12(1):39–48.

13. West TA, Rush SM. Total talus replacement: case series and literature review. J Foot Ankle Surg 2021;60(1):187–93.

Updates of Total Ankle Replacement Revision Options

New Generation Total Ankle Replacement Revision Options, Stemmed Implants, Peri-Articular Osteotomies

Vincent G. Vacketta, DPM, AACFAS[a],[*],
Jacob M. Perkins, DPM, AACFAS[a], Christoper F. Hyer, DPM, MS, FACFAS[a]

KEYWORDS

- Ankle arthritis • Total ankle replacement • Revision surgery • Deformity correction

KEY POINTS

- Thorough clinical, radiographic, and laboratory workup is critical to understand the cause of primary TAR failure and allow for appropriate revision planning and patient optimization before revision TAR.
- Osseous considerations for revision TAR include restoration of joint alignment perpendicular to the mechanical axis of the limb, use of bone grafting or metal augments when necessary, and correction of any extra-articular pedal or proximal deformity before or at the time of implantation.
- Soft tissue considerations for revision TAR include neutralize ankle through soft-tissue balancing via repair, reconstruction, or sequential soft tissue release and establish a medial or later "tether-point" to serve as a frontal plane axis of rotation for soft tissue balancing.
- When selecting revision TAR implant, one should select an implant, which provides the greatest stability through the tibial component as well as through the articulation of the talar and polyethelene componentry. When possible, the implant selected should bridge across any cystic or compromised bone in order to seat the implant in healthier viable bone.
- Staging should be considered when significant osseous or soft tissue rebalancing is required.

[a] Orthopedic Foot and Ankle Center, 350 West Wilson Bridge Road, Suite 200, Worthington, OH 43085, USA
* Corresponding author.
E-mail address: vvacketta@gmail.com

Clin Podiatr Med Surg 40 (2023) 749–767
https://doi.org/10.1016/j.cpm.2023.05.015
0891-8422/23/© 2023 Elsevier Inc. All rights reserved.

INTRODUCTION

Ankle arthritis is a disabling disease pattern resulting in pain and dysfunction ultimately leading to a reduction in quality of life. Unlike more common arthritides of the knee and hip, ankle arthritis is unique in its presentation with an earlier onset of end-stage disease and an etiology, which is most-commonly posttraumatic in nature.[1,2] Due to the higher prevalence of young and active individuals within this patient population, a concerted effort has been made to develop and improve total ankle prosthesis in order to improve quality of life in this young population and prevent further degeneration of the surrounding joints.

Through continued research and design, improvements have continued to be made as newer generation implants are developed. Recent studies evaluating the newest fourth-generation implants have shown promising results although long-term studies are still lacking.[3–6] Although long-term studies on the newer third-generation and fourth-generation implants leave much to be desired, long-term follow-up of the older generation implants have demonstrated the need for revision surgery.[7–11] These results have inspired several manufacturers to focus their efforts not only on the development of primary prosthesis but also on the development of revision implants. The advent of true revision total ankle replacement (TAR) systems have allowed for more complex deformity and pathology to be addressed as well as for primary TAR to be done in patients aged younger than 50 years who might overlast the primary implant and need revision later in life. This article discusses the considerations for revision TAR based on the current revision options and a treatment algorithm developed by the lead author.

CLINICAL PRESENTATION

Before consideration of revision surgery, thorough evaluation and proper patient workup is required to fully understand the cause and mechanism of the implant failure. Clinical evaluation should include a thorough evaluation of the patient, unshod, in both static stance as well as a comprehensive gait analysis. Particular attention should be given to the overall alignment of the limb to assess for concomitant knee, hip, or spinopelvic deformity, which may significantly alter the mechanical axis of the limb. A thorough vascular and neurologic examination should be performed to rule out any vascular or neurologic deficits. If abnormalities are present, additional testing or consultation should be implemented to allow for further assessment and possible preoperative optimization. The soft tissue envelope should be thoroughly evaluated for earlier surgical incisions, potential adhesion, and signs of venous or arterial compromise. The underlying soft tissue structures should be examined for the presence of pain, weakness, or contractures such as equinus, which may limit the appropriate function of the implant. Utilization of seated range of motion assessment may be beneficial in elucidating more subtle soft tissue pathologic condition, which may limit the appropriate range of motion. Appropriate evaluation of the hindfoot, midfoot, and forefoot position are also imperative to evaluate any underlying deformity, which may be affecting the function of the prosthesis. The use of diagnostic injections may also be beneficial in further understanding the cause of the patient's pain if peri-implant or adjacent joint pathologic condition is suspected.

DIAGNOSTIC IMAGING

Imaging plays an important role in both understanding the potential causes of implant failure as well as providing information for operative planning. A complete and bilateral radiographic assessment should be performed, consisting of standardized weight-bearing anterior–posterior and lateral radiographs of the ankle and foot. Bilateral long-leg axial views are also recommended to evaluate for any valgus or varus deformity and to evaluate potential prosthetic migration and bone loss. A computed tomography (CT) scan, preferably weight-bearing with metal subtraction protocol, can be an additional tool to further assess for cystic changes, overall bone quality, osseointegration, and the presence of periprosthetic arthritis. This imaging modality is particularly useful in instances where the talar component design impedes appropriate evaluation of the underlying osseous structure on plain film radiographs. Additional imaging modalities such as single-photon emission CT (SPECT) may be beneficial in identifying pathologic processes around the TAR components such as aseptic loosening or gutter impingement.

LABORATORY VALUES

As with any failed orthopedic joint implant, prosthetic joint infection (PJI) must be ruled out. After evaluating for any obvious signs of deep infection on physical examination, one should implement a thorough laboratory evaluation consisting of erythrocyte sedimentation rate (ESR), C-reactive protein (CRP), procalcitonin, and complete blood count (CBC) with differential. Additionally, serum interleukin-6 has 97% accuracy and 100% specificity in the identification of periprosthetic infections.[12] Elevation or abnormality in any of the aforementioned laboratory values warrants further confirmation via joint aspiration for synovial fluid analysis and analysis of synovial alpha-defensin. Indium-labeled tagged WBC scan may serve as another useful modality for evaluation if PJI is suspected.

REVISION ARTHROPLASTY, ARTHRODESIS, OR AMPUTATION

After meticulous evaluation and determination of the cause of implant failure, thorough consultation with the patient and family is imperative. Although significant advancements have improved the efficacy of revision TAR, one must realize that this option may not always be in the best interest of the parties involved. Additional revision options for TAR include conversion to arthrodesis or amputation, both of which have their own inherent advantages, disadvantages, and risks, which must be thoroughly communicated to the patient. When determining the most appropriate path for revision, a well-established and pragmatic treatment algorithm can be a beneficial tool in guiding the surgeon toward the most suitable revision option for the patient scenario.

CAUSE AND TREATMENT OF PRIMARY TOTAL ANKLE REPLACEMENT FAILURE

As mentioned previously, the cause and indications for revision TAR are broad, and as such, the approach to revision TAR must be individualized and case specific. Again, utilizing an established treatment algorithm can significantly benefit the surgeon in determining the most appropriate approach for revision TAR.

ASEPTIC LOOSENING AND SUBSIDENCE

Aseptic loosening with or without subsidence in TAR can occur due to several causes including periprosthetic osteolysis, avascular necrosis, component migration, and malalignment.[13] Understanding the cause of aseptic loosening is critical to ensure appropriate selection of revision procedures. Selection of revision TAR components may also be altered, depending on which side component experienced loosening and if any significant bone loss or defect has resulted.

COMPONENT MIGRATION

Component migration is a physiologic process occurring within the first months of TAR and must be closely monitored for progression and symptomatology. Patients who exhibit component migration are at risk for early TAR failure, and the decision for revision TAR is determined by patient pain and integrity of the underlying osseous integrity.[14] Component migration, which lacks continued progression and is asymptomatic, may be closely monitored without the need for revision TAR.

AVASCULAR NECROSIS

Avascular necrosis can be a devastating complication, which may occur on the tibial or talar surfaces and result in periprosthetic osteolysis and subsequent component subsidence. Osseointegration is a predominant factor in component stability and longevity, which is significantly compromised in the setting of avascular, necrotic bone.

Management of talar avascular necrosis in TAR is determined largely by the extent of subsidence and the amount of viable talus remaining. In the setting of minimal subsidence and viable talar bone stock, revision TAR may be performed with resection of avascular bone until healthy talus is encountered. A "flat top" talus design is preferred in this setting with supplementary fixation as needed in order to provide a stable cortical surface for implant setting and osseointegration. Adjunctive subtalar joint arthrodesis may also be considered if the proximity of the resection margin is near the subtalar joint. In the setting of severe avascular necrosis, subsidence, and osteolysis, a customized total talus prosthesis may be considered. Several recent studies have shown favorable short-term outcomes using this salvage option in the setting of severe talar subsidence secondary to avascular necrosis.[15,16]

PERIPROSTHETIC CYSTS

Periprosthetic cyst formation can present similar complications to those seen in patients with aseptic loosening and subsidence and can often be the cause of the aforementioned complications if not appropriately addressed. The formation of periprosthetic cyst is one that is not completely understood, although several plausible theories exist.[17–22] Regardless of their cause, periprosthetic cysts must be closely monitored to evaluate for progression. Routine plain film radiographs should be obtained to monitor cyst progression. Cysts that are large, are in close proximity to the prosthesis, or show progression should also be evaluated using CT, which has been shown to be superior in the evaluation of periprosthetic cysts.[17] In addition to plain film radiographs and CT, SPECT can be a beneficial clinical tool in determining the stability of the implant in relation to the cyst formation.

Conservative monitoring versus surgical management of cyst formation is greatly determined by location, size, and progression of the cyst. In regards to location, cysts within the talus are considered to be more concerning for implant complications due to the limited bone stock of the talus when compared with the tibia. A classification system developed by Berlet and colleagues serves as a comprehensive classification system for evaluating talar cyst formation on CT scan and provides insightful recommendations for management based on cyst size, location, and progression. Cyst location is also relevant in regards to the proximity to the prosthesis. Cysts that communicate with the bone-prosthesis interface can easily compromise the stability of the prosthesis leading to subsidence and failure.

The importance of size and progression of the periprosthetic cyst also largely depends on location. Cysts that are in close proximity to the implant or cortical bone must be monitored more closely as progression or significant cyst size may lead to the loss of implant stability or periarticular fracture. Several studies have evaluated the size of periprosthetic cysts in attempts to quantify cysts, which require surgical intervention versus close monitoring.[17–22] Although these studies have provided valuable insight to cyst management, no consensus has been reached in regards to the need for intervention based on cyst size.[17–22] The senior author initiates surgical management on periprosthetic cysts that are greater than 1 cm in their largest diameter and have documented evidence of progression.

The decision to proceed with TAR revision lies predominantly of the size, location, and progressive nature of the cyst, whereas the presence of pain or symptoms associated with the periprosthetic cyst or cysts remains less relevant in the determination of surgical management versus conservative monitoring. In the absence of pain or symptoms, cysts that are of significant size, show progression, or are in close proximity to the implant are managed surgically by the senior author in an effort to preserve implant stability.

When surgical intervention is warranted, the decision to perform simple bone grafting versus component revision is highly determined by the stability of the prosthesis. Although the use of SPECT provides valuable insight between the probability of loosening on imaging and intraoperative findings, the intraoperative assessment of remaining bone stock and implant stability following cyst debridement remains an important determinant for component revision versus grafting.

When compromised implant stability and poor remaining bone stock require implant revision, one must be cognizant to maintain the appropriate joint line to ensure appropriate function of the revision implant. Preoperative planning with the use of bony landmarks for reference as described by Harnroongroj can aid the surgeon intraoperatively visualizing the native joint line during revision surgery.[23] In mild-to-moderate tibial metaphyseal bone loss restoration of the joint line can be achieved through impaction bone grafting. The authors routinely use a medullary stemmed implant for these revision cases because this design allows for "bridging" across the cystic bone into healthier more stable bone proximally. Additionally this design inherently provides more stability than other minimal resection, resurfacing-type implants that engage the tibia with smaller keels, pegs, or fins.

In the case of significant tibial metaphyseal bone loss, the use of modular metaphyseal componentry can be beneficial for metallic augmentation of distal tibia bone loss. This concept, which has been extrapolated from revision total knee arthroplasty, produces a stable platform to reestablish the native joint line. In instances where the revised joint line remains proximal to the native joint line after maximizing the metal augment length, the surgeon may further migrate the joint line distally through increasing the size of the polyethylene component. Sizing of the polyethylene component should be performed so that the distal extent of the polyethylene is in line with the native arthritic ankle joint line.

MALALIGNMENT

A critical component in achieving successful outcomes with total ankle arthroplasty relies on the ability to implant the prosthesis appropriately along the mechanical axis of the limb. This task can become particularly challenging in instances of significant congenital, developmental, or posttraumatic deformity.

Any form of malalignment, whether driven by deformity or due to technique error, will significantly jeopardize the long-term viability of the prosthesis. In cases of TAR failure due to malalignment, the assessment must be holistic and evaluate not only the local site of failure but also the alignment of the lower limb from toes to hip. Any evidence of proximal deformity must be addressed before or at the time of revision TAR. In the instance of deformity at the proximal third of the tibia, knee, femur, or hip leading to TAR failure, deformity correction should be pursued before revision TAR as is recommended before primary TAR. If proximal deformity correction is performed following primary or revision TAR, the probability of further revision TAR surgery is large due to the changes in lower limb mechanical axis. Utilizing the center of rotation axis to guide deformity correction, the treatment of extra-articular deformity can be treated through various wedge or dome osteotomies and may be performed concomitantly with revision TAR or in a staged fashion.[24,25] In addition, when a stable implant is present, reports have shown favorable outcomes performing isolated tibial osteotomies for frontal plane correction without revision of the implant.[25]

Equally important to the management of proximal deformity, one must ensure that the foot is without deformity beneath the ankle. Unrecognized or unaddressed pedal deformity can be a significant risk factor for TAR failure even when implant selection and placement is appropriate. The decision to perform pedal correction in a staged fashion or simultaneously with primary or revision TAR is based on surgeon experience and the nature of the corrective procedures performed. Ultimately, malalignment of TAR can occur in all planes because of extra-articular or intra-articular deformity, each with its own unique considerations. The remainder of this article will review the unique considerations for revision TAR deformity that is intra-articular in nature.

FRONTAL PLANE MALALIGNMENT

When evaluating frontal plane deformity in TAR, whether primary or revision TAR, one must first establish the congruency of the tibiotalar joint. Whether varus or valgus, deformities with greater than $10°$ difference between tibial and talar joint lines are considered incongruent, and those with less than $10°$ difference are considered congruent. Congruent deformities tend to be driven primarily by osseous deformity, whereas incongruent deformities often result from significant soft tissue imbalances or a combination of both soft tissue and osseous pathologic condition.

CONGRUENT DEFORMITY REVISION TOTAL ANKLE REPLACEMENT

Similar concepts apply to managing congruent deformity TAR failures, as when managing congruent deformity in primary TAR. Failure in this instance stems from malalignment of the primary implant, which can lead to a multitude of complications such as edge-loading, stress-shielding, and aseptic loosening. Congruent deformity in TAR often results from inadequate correction of a congruent deformity with primary implant or can be iatrogenic through malaligned coupled cuts during primary TAR. This can be a relatively easy mistake to occur especially in cases of preexisting tibial varum. For the purpose of this discussion, deformities secondary to component subsidence will be excluded. Revision TAR in the congruent ankle can commonly be performed in a single-stage fashion. The primary goal of revision surgery in these cases is to reestablish the joint line perpendicular to the mechanical axis of the lower extremity. This results in a biased or wedged cut, most commonly in the tibia, which will correct the angular deformity of the joint line and bring the ankle into a more neutral position in reference to the mechanical axis of the limb. After correction is achieved with osseous cuts, the ankle should be reevaluated for stability with the trial implant in place to ensure that no soft tissue imbalance remains. If present, any soft tissue imbalances should be corrected via ligament reconstruction or controlled sequential release or a combination of the two.

INCONGRUENT DEFORMITY REVISION TOTAL ANKLE REPLACEMENT

TAR deformities that are greater than 10° of angulation between tibial and talar component joint axes are considered incongruent. These deformities are most commonly a result of soft tissue imbalance but can also be osseous in nature. As mentioned previously, for the purpose of this discussion, deformities secondary to component subsidence will be excluded. In contrast to congruent deformity in revision TAR, the likelihood of requiring a staged approach is more common when significant soft tissue imbalance is present. Staging is more common in the incongruent valgus revision than in the incongruent varus revision TAR. When managing soft tissue imbalance in TAR, one must attempt to "tether" the ankle to a medial or lateral constraint and develop the opposite side of the joint off of this tether point.

In the instance of a varus ankle, the medial soft tissues are contracted and the lateral soft tissues are attenuated or damaged. Through reconstruction, the lateral ligament tension is restored and serves as a tether point when performing the subsequent sequential release of the medial soft tissue structures. Due to the reproducibility and consistent results achieved with lateral ankle ligament reconstruction, incongruent varus deformity in TAR is therefore more amenable to be performed in a single-stage fashion. **Figs. 1–6** represent a case series demonstrating a revision TAR in an incongruent varus ankle with revision to a medullary stemmed implant and hindfoot realignment via posterior calcaneal osteotomy.

In a valgus incongruent TAR revision, the same concepts apply though the tether point is created through the deltoid ligament and balancing occurs through the lateral ankle ligament complex. The success of primary or revision TAR in the valgus deformity lies heavily on the integrity of the deltoid ligament. Intraoperatively one must determine viability of the deltoid ligament as well as its respective "end-point" where the ligament regains tension. In cases where the deltoid ligament has a discernible endpoint and can be used as a viable tether point, rebalancing and revision is performed through sequential lateral release until the ankle joint is balanced to neutral. If a neutral ankle is achieved with adequate soft tissue constraints then revision TAR

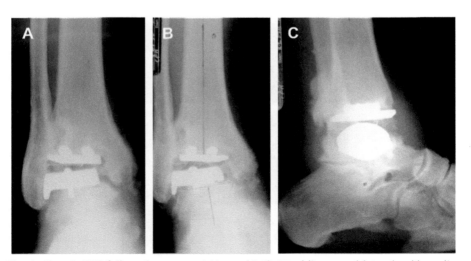

Fig. 1. Case 1: TAR failure: incongruent Varus. (*A–C*) AP, oblique, and lateral ankle radiographs demonstrating mobile-bearing TAR failure with incongruent varus deformity, osteolysis, and cyst formation.

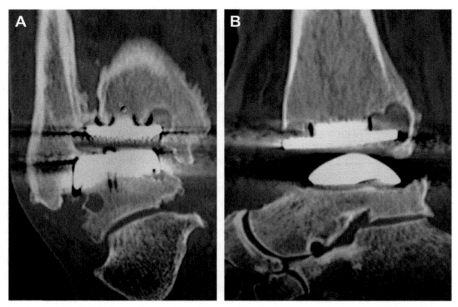

Fig. 2. Case 1: TAR failure: incongruent Varus. (*A*, *B*) CT images demonstrating cyst formation surrounding tibial and talar components.

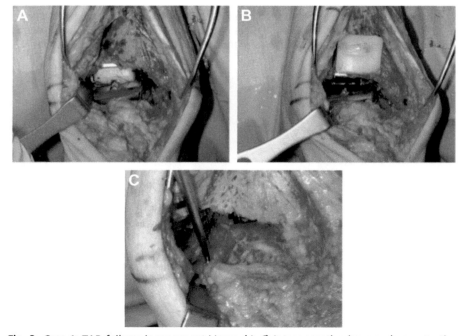

Fig. 3. Case 1: TAR failure: incongruent Varus. (*A–C*) Intraoperative images demonstrating implant subsidence and underlying cysts following explantation.

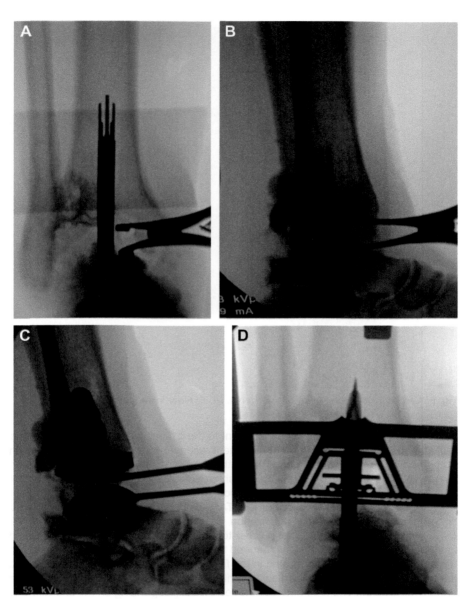

Fig. 4. Case 1: TAR failure: incongruent Varus. (*A–D*) Intraoperative fluoroscopy demonstrating reduction and tibial and talar preparation and trial implants. Note, the ankle is reduced to neutral with a lamina spreader to allow for the use of coupled cuts.

implantation is performed. In addition to revision with a medullary stemmed implant, some additional stability can be afforded through the use of a larger polyethylene component and utilizing an implant with a sulcus-type talar component.

In instances where complete deltoid tear or attenuation is present and no end-point exists, then reconstruction must be performed to create a viable tether for lateral ligament balancing. Several various deltoid ligament reconstructions have been described

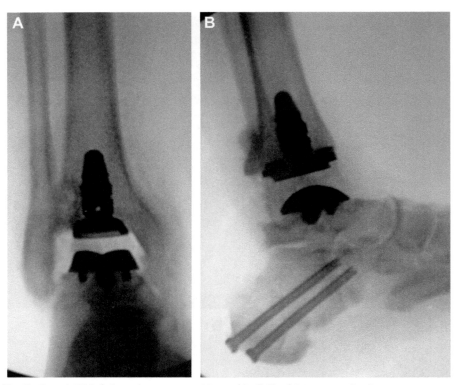

Fig. 5. Case 1: TAR failure: incongruent Varus. (*A, B*) Final intraoperative images.

in the literature, which serves as a testament to the difficulties in developing a consistent and reproducible method for this ligament reconstruction. Due to the inconsistent outcomes with this reconstruction, the authors prefer to perform these incongruent valgus TAR and revision TAR in a staged fashion to allow for the assessment of the deltoid ligament before the staged TAR revision. Traditionally, the first stage of revision TAR in this scenario consists of primary TAR explant, deltoid ligament reconstruction/augmentation, and ankle stabilization via utilization of a cement spacer within the lateral aspect of the ankle joint in order to stabilize the ankle into a neutral position. Finally, any osteotomies or fusions required to establish a neutral and well-aligned foot beneath the ankle will be performed in the first stage of revision TAR. Realignment of the foot beneath the ankle is particularly critical in the setting of valgus TAR, whether primary or revision. The time between stages will vary depending on the ancillary procedures performed. In instances where additional fusion or osteotomies are required in the initial stage, the authors will confirm consolidation at 10 to 12 weeks postoperatively via WBCT before proceeding with the second stage. If failure of the first stage occurs, particularly in regards to the deltoid ligament and medial constraints, one should strongly consider conversion to arthrodesis. Once consolidation of both the soft tissue and osseous reconstructions has been established, second-stage revision TAR can be performed. During implantation, care must be taken to implant the prosthesis in alignment with the mechanical axis of the lower extremity because alignment becomes increasingly critical with revision TAR. Equally important is the soft tissue balancing, particularly in the incongruent valgus TAR and evaluation on medial and lateral soft

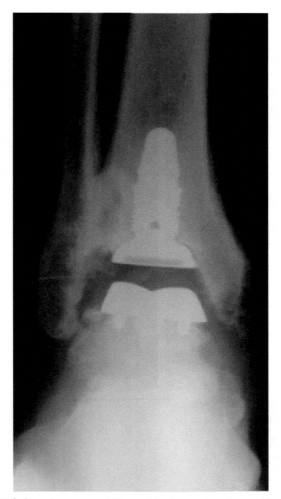

Fig. 6. Case 1: TAR failure: incongruent Varus. Most recent postoperative radiograph.

tissue constraints should be performed before initial cuts, when trialing, and following final implantation. In contrast to the revision varus TAR, the tether point in valgus TAR becomes the deltoid ligament and balancing of the ankle should primarily be performed through sequential release or reconstruction of the lateral ankle ligaments in order to achieve a neutral ankle. **Figs. 7–11** represent a case series demonstrating a staged primary TAR in an incongruent valgus ankle with subsequent revision secondary to aseptic loosening and osteolysis.

SAGITTAL PLANE MALALIGNMENT

Similar to malalignment in the frontal plane, sagittal plane malalignment can result in TAR dysfunction and failure. Malalignment in this scenario often results from overcorrection or undercorrection of deformity with primary implant or can be iatrogenic through malaligned cuts during primary TAR. Malalignment in the sagittal plane can result in anterior or posterior subluxation of the talus beneath the tibia resulting in

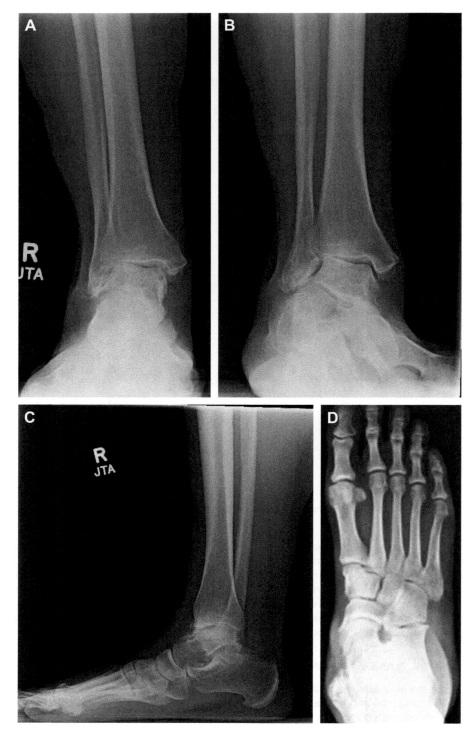

Fig. 7. Case 2: Incongruent Valgus, Staged, Revision. (*A–D*) Preoperative radiographs demonstrating incongruent ankle valgus and progressive collapsing foot deformity.

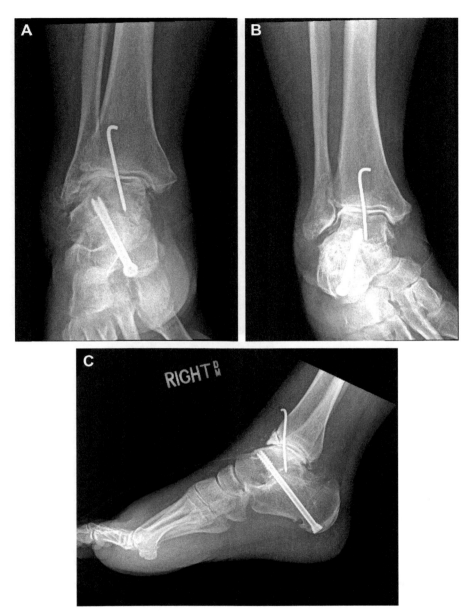

Fig. 8. Case 2: Incongruent Valgus, Staged, Revision. (*A–C*) Postoperative radiographs demonstrating stage 1: Reconstruction with subtalar joint arthrodesis, posterior calcaneal osteotomy, and deltoid reconstruction with intra-articular cement spacer.

either increased instability or limitations in range of motion. When evaluating TAR failure in the sagittal plane, it is important to delineate between soft tissue and osseous causes. Posterior capsule adhesion, gastrocnemius or gastrocsoleus equinus, and/or overlengthening of the posterior muscle group can be common causes of sagittal

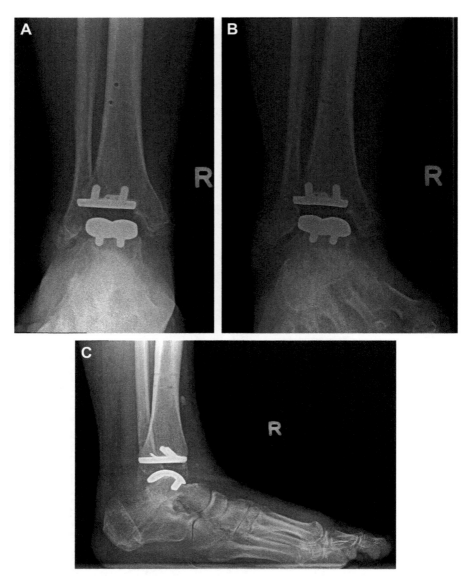

Fig. 9. Case 2: Incongruent Valgus, Staged, Revision. (*A–C*) Postoperative radiographs demonstrating stage 2: Hardware removal with TAR.

plane dysfunction, which can be addressed with relatively minor procedures not requiring revision TAR. Revision TAR due to sagittal plane malalignment weighs more heavily on the alignment of the osseous cuts rather than soft tissue balancing as seen in correcting frontal plane malalignment. The slope of the tibial and talar cuts should be made perpendicular to the weight-bearing axis of the lower extremity. In instances where excessive anterior or posterior subluxation of the talus is present, cuts can be performed with some bias toward posterior or anterior slope in order to better position the talus beneath the tibia. If TAR failure occurs due to excessive

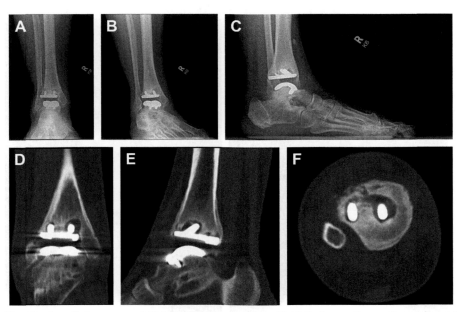

Fig. 10. Case 2: Incongruent Valgus, Staged, Revision. (*A–F*) Postoperative radiographs and CT demonstrating: osteolysis and lucency surrounding tibial component.

posterior or anterior slope, then revision cuts should be performed on a bias in order to establish the appropriate joint line with respect to the mechanical axis of the limb. Considerations must be given to limb shortening with tibial cuts and proximity to the subtalar joint with corrective cuts on the talus. In instances of significant bone loss due to corrective cuts, the use of modular metaphyseal componentry can be beneficial for metallic augmentation of distal tibia bone loss and similar metallic augments exist for the talus with some manufacturers.

Implant Selection

Prosthesis selection revision TAR is critical in achieving a successful revision outcome. With advancements in TAR technology, many companies now offer revision components, which can serve as adequate revision options. Often due to the nature of revision surgery, the native bone stock and soft tissue constraint is relatively poor when compared with primary procedures. Due to these realities, the ideal implant should be one that is constrained, provides intrinsic stability, and is able to bridge and integrate past the earlier site of TAR implantation. In order to extend past the primary TAR footprint, the senior author often uses a modular stemmed tibial component, which affords more stability when compared with other implant designs. In addition, the modular aspect of the component allows for the surgeon to increase the working length of the implant on an as-needed basis. At a minimum, if low-profile resurfacing type tibial components are used for revision, the tibial fixation should be different from the primary implant and increase stability in some fashion.

In regards to talar implants, the senior author prefers a "flat-top" talus design, which allows for the implant to sit on the stable cortical rim of the talus. The senior author also uses additional modular base componentry when necessary allowing for more of the implant to rest on cortical bone, again providing further stability. The author prefers

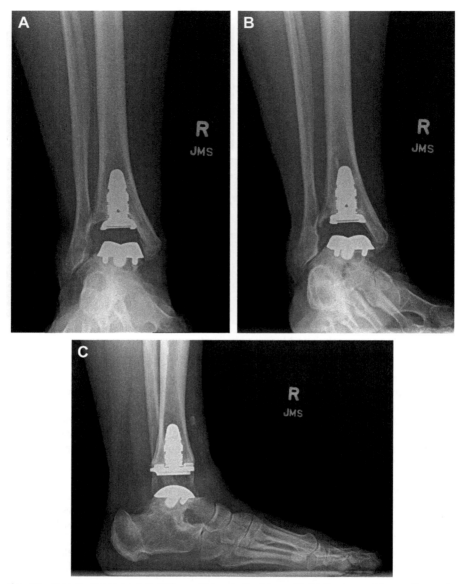

Fig. 11. Case 2: Incongruent Valgus, Staged, Revision. (A–C) Postoperative radiographs demonstrating revision TAR with medullary stemmed tibial component and flat-top sulcus-type talus component.

talar components, which have a sulcus-type interface with the polyethylene, which provides additional constraint and stability to the implant. As mentioned previously, if talar bone stock is not sufficient to support a revision talar component, total talar replacement prostheses serves as an acceptable revision talar component. The polyethylene component should be fixed bearing and in an effort to appropriately tension the adjacent soft tissues, the lead author will often increase polyethylene thickness when appropriate.

SUMMARY

Developments in research and technology have allowed for advancements in the methods and modalities for the treatment of ankle arthritis, particularly with TAR. As with any orthopedic prosthesis, complications, revisions, and failures occur with TAR, and the ability to manage these outcomes is a necessary skill set for any arthroplasty surgeon. The importance of thorough clinical evaluation and patient optimization is a crucial aspect of managing TAR complications and patient expectations, which cannot be overlooked. Clinical and radiographic assessments must be correlated in order to diagnose and appropriately address the complications at hand. By understanding the cause of the complication or failure, one may then devise the next appropriate treatment options for the patient. In instances of failure, one must understand when salvage is achievable and whether staged revision is necessary. Along with thorough clinical and radiographic evaluation, operative treatment must be well thought out, and communication with all members of the operative team is critical for a successful outcome with minimal intraoperative setbacks. Imparting the recommendations in this article, one should approach revision TAR with the aim to restore soft tissue balance, manage osseous deficits, reestablish the native joint line with modular components or grafting as needed, and use implants that impart the greatest level of stability.

CLINICS CARE POINTS

- Ankle arthritis is a condition, which affects approximately 2% to 5% of the population and is most commonly a sequela of earlier trauma.

- The ongoing developments of TAR systems, both primary and revision, have lead to an expansion in the utilization and applications of TAR in ankle arthritis and deformity.

- The approach to revision TAR begins with thorough evaluation and clinical workup including: extensive physical examination, static stance and gait analysis, weight-bearing radiographs and appropriate advanced imaging, as well as necessary laboratory values. One must ascertain the cause of primary TAR failure before consideration of revision TAR.

- Surgical principles for revision TAR include the following:
  o Osseous correction: Reestablish a joint alignment perpendicular to the mechanical axis of the limb, reestablish joint height with use of bone grafting or metal augments when necessary, select implants which will provide stability and span across poorer quality bone when present, stage when appropriate.
  o Soft tissue correction: Balance soft tissues to establish a neutral ankle through repair, reconstruction, or soft tissue release, establish a stable "tether-point" to balance the ankle, stage when appropriate.

DISCLOSURE

No funding was received for this publication, and there are no conflicts of interest.

REFERENCES

1. Saltzman CL, Salamon ML, Blanchard M, et al. Saltzman epidemiology ankle arthritis. JBJS. Iowa Orthopeadic J. 2005;25:44–6.
2. SooHoo NF, Zingmond DS, Ko CY. Comparison of reoperationrates following ankle arthrodesis and total ankle arthroplasty. J Bone Joint Surg Am 2007; 89(10):2143–9.

3. Rushing CJ, Zulauf E, Hyer CF, et al. Risk factors for early failure of fourth generation total ankle arthroplasty prostheses. J Foot Ankle Surg 2021;60(2):312–7. Epub 2020 Oct 16. PMID: 33168439.

4. Rushing CJ, Kibbler K, Hyer CF, et al. The INFINITY total ankle prosthesis: outcomes at short-term follow-up. Foot Ankle Spec 2022;15(2):119–26. PMID: 32772552.

5. Rushing CJ, Law R, Hyer CF. Early experience with the CADENCE total ankle prosthesis. J Foot Ankle Surg 2021;60(1):67–73. Epub 2020 Sep 1. PMID: 33129676.

6. Rushing CJ, Mckenna BJ, Zulauf EA, et al. Intermediate-term outcomes of a third-generation, 2-component total ankle prosthesis. Foot Ankle Int 2021;42(7): 935–43. PMID: 33508961.

7. Cody EA, Taylor MA, Nunley JA, et al. Increased early revision rate with the INFINITY total ankle prosthesis. Foot Ankle Int 2019;40(1):9–17.

8. Roukis TS. Incidence of revision after primary implantation of the Agility™ total ankle replacement system: a systematic review. J Foot Ankle Surg 2012;51(2): 198–204.

9. Buechel FF, Buechel FF, Pappas MJ. Twenty-year evaluation of cementless mobile-bearing total ankle replacements. Clin Orthop Relat Res 2004;424:19–26.

10. Groth HE, Fitch HF. Salvage procedures for complications of total ankle arthroplasty. Clin Orthop Relat Res 1987;224:244–50.

11. Henricson A, Carlsson A, Rydholm U. What is a revision of total ankle replacement? Foot Ankle Surg 2011;17(3):99–102.

12. Di Cesare PE, Chang E, Preston CF, et al. Serum interleukin-6 as a marker of periprosthetic infection following total hip and knee arthroplasty. J Bone Joint Surg Am 2005;87(9):1921–7. PMID: 16140805.

13. Li SY, Myerson MS. Management of talar component subsidence. Foot Ankle Clin 2017;22(2):361–89.

14. Dunbar MJ, Fong JW, Wilson DA, et al. Longitudinal migration and inducible displacement of the mobility total ankle system. Acta Orthop 2012;83(4):394–400.

15. West TA, Rush SM. Total talus replacement: case series and literature review. J Foot Ankle Surg 2021;60(1):187–93. Epub 2020 Aug 26. PMID: 33218861.

16. Angthong C. Anatomic total talar prosthesis replacement surgery and ankle arthroplasty: an early case series in Thailand. Orthop Rev 2014;6(3):5486.

17. Yoon HS, Lee J, Choi WJ, et al. Periprosthetic osteolysis after total ankle arthroplasty. Foot Ankle Int 2014;35(1):14–21.

18. Schipper ON, Haddad SL, Pytel P, et al. Histological analysis of early osteolysis in total ankle arthroplasty. Foot Ankle Int 2017;38(4):351–9.

19. Berlet GC, Penner MJ, Prissel MA, et al. CT-based descriptive classification for residual talar defects associated with failed total ankle replacement: technique tip. Foot Ankle Int 2018;39(5):568–72.

20. Rodriguez D, Bevernage BD, Maldague P, et al. Medium term follow-up of the AES ankle prosthesis: high rate of asymptomatic osteolysis. Foot Ankle Surg 2010;16(2):54–60.

21. Pyevich MT, Saltzman CL, Callaghan JJ, et al. Total ankle arthroplasty: a unique design. Two to twelve-year follow-up. J Bone Joint Surg Am 1998;80(10): 1410–20.

22. Johansson L, Edlund U, Fahlgren A, et al. Bone resorption induced by fluid flow. J Biomech Eng 2009;131(9):094505.

23. Harnroongroj T, Hummel A, Ellis SJ, et al. Assessing the ankle joint line level before and after total ankle arthroplasty with the "Joint Line Height Ratio". Foot Ankle Orthop 2019;4(4). 247301141988435.
24. DeOrio JK. Total ankle replacements with malaligned ankles: osteotomies performed simultaneously with TAA. Foot Ankle Int 2012;33(4):344–6.
25. Deforth M, Kr.henbuhl N, Zwicky L, et al. Supramalleolar osteotomy for tibial component malposition in total ankle replacement. Foot Ankle Int 2017;38(9): 952–6.

The Role of Supramalleolar Osteotomies in Ankle Arthritis

Sara Mateen, DPM[a], Noman A. Siddiqui, DPM, MHA[a,b,*]

KEYWORDS

- Joint preservation • Subtalar joint • Tibial procurvatum • Tibial recurvatum
- Total ankle arthroplasty • Valgus ankle • Varus ankle

KEY POINTS

- Comprehend basic deformity correction principles as they pertain to the supramalleolar osteotomy by realigning the mechanical axis for improved weight distribution through the ankle joint.
- Appreciate the literature in terms of surgical considerations with respect to ankle arthritis with staged and concomitant procedures for deformity correction.
- Understand preoperative clinical and radiographic work-up before the supramalleolar osteotomy with an update on advanced imaging to help determine the effects of the supramalleolar osteotomy on overall joint alignment.

INTRODUCTION

Over 90% of ankle osteoarthritis (OA) is secondary to trauma.[1] The condition's post-traumatic etiology can cause deformity to occur in both the coronal (valgus or varus) and sagittal (procurvatum or recurvatum) planes.[2–7] The ankle joint carries relatively four times the body's weight during the stance phase of gait, all within a scant contact area consisting of approximately 522 mm,[8] which is 33% of the hip and knee joints.[9] The ankle joint can withstand greater tensile and shear forces than the hip and knee joint despite greater contact pressures with thinner cartilage.[10] Owing to the posttraumatic nature of ankle arthritis and its uneven stresses across the joint surface, patients frequently become symptomatic earlier when compared with cases of degenerative primary OA of the hip and knee joints. This earlier onset underscores the importance of joint-preserving options.[6,9,11]

[a] International Center of Limb Lengthening, Rubin Institute of Advanced Orthopedics, 2401 West Belvedere Avenue, Baltimore, MD 21215, USA; [b] Division of Podiatry, Sinai and Northwest Hospital, 2401 West Belvedere Avenue, Baltimore, MD 21215, USA
* Corresponding author.
E-mail address: siddiqui.dpm@gmail.com

Clin Podiatr Med Surg 40 (2023) 769–781
https://doi.org/10.1016/j.cpm.2023.05.017
0891-8422/23/© 2023 Elsevier Inc. All rights reserved.

Joint-preserving procedures are one of two main methods of surgical management for ankle arthritis (the other being joint-sacrificing). The joint-preserving category includes ankle arthroscopy with debridement, distraction arthroplasty, osteochondral defect management, and corrective supramalleolar osteotomies (SMOs). Joint-sacrificing procedures would include either ankle arthrodesis or total ankle arthroplasty (TAA).[8] Surgical work-up can be elaborated further via primary osseous malalignment (with or without ligamentous insufficiency) or primary ligamentous malalignment (with or without secondary osseous malalignment). It is important not only to address the ankle joint but also the adjacent structures when planning for correction.[8,9]

The SMO is a joint-preserving surgical procedure that allows realignment of the ankle joint in severe deformity secondary to arthritis.[12-16] This osteotomy realigns the mechanical axis to provide better weight distribution through the ankle joint. With an aligned mechanical axis, the overloaded asymmetric ankle joint will shift toward the preserved joint area in a valgus or varus ankle joint. The SMO also can be used via a staged approach to correct severe deformity in an end-stage arthritic ankle before TAA to optimize the implant's longevity and improve overall functional outcomes.[17-19]

The SMO is a potent surgical approach for joint preservation. In addition to OA, SMOs may be used for congenital or acquired developmental deformities, malunited distal tibia fractures, and malunited ankle fusions.[15] Like any technique, a complete understanding of deformity correction and full patient work-up—both clinically and radiographically—are necessary for optimal patient outcomes,[16] alongside meticulous preoperative planning and precise execution in the operating room. Variations of the SMO approach exist to correct varus, valgus, procurvatum, and recurvatum deformities of the distal tibia. Similarly, there are multiple fixation methods, including gradual or acute correction and internal or external fixation. The present study aims to provide an overview of SMO use in OA correction for varus, valgus, procurvatum, and recuravatum deformities.

PREOPERATIVE CLINICAL EVALUATION

Regarding OA correction, it is essential to be concerned not only with correcting osseous malalignment but also ligamentous compromise. Many patients with asymmetric ankle arthritis demonstrate instability of the ankle joint, adjacent joints, and/or stabilizing soft tissue structures.[20,21] Ankle valgus often is well tolerated due to a greater amount of inversion compensation available at the subtalar joint (STJ). However, if no STJ motion is available, patients may develop first ray symptoms.[15] A careful clinical examination is necessary to examine these structures and determine whether additional procedures are warranted.

Muscle and tendon contracture should be examined preoperatively, including conducting a Silfverskiold test of the ankle joint in knee extension and flexion to determine gastrocnemius or gastrocnemius-solus equinus.[15] A weight-bearing assessment of the patient is recommended to evaluate for any compensation with ankle deformity and subsequent effect upon gait.[15] In addition to coronal plane instability, the talus may be extruded anteriorly out of the mortise, causing further subtalar malalignment and segmental deformity, which will need to be addressed.[20,21]

A fixed deformity of the distal tibia can cause compensatory deformity within the foot and ankle. For example, if distal tibial varus was corrected by SMO without thorough clinical evaluation, the foot may be left in a valgus position due to an unobserved STJ eversion contracture.[15] To examine for this, place the foot in a maximum deformity position—if this cannot be achieved, a fixed compensatory contracture exists.

Contraindications for SMO may be observed in the thorough clinical evaluation. Hindfoot instability is a major consideration and SMO surgery should not occur if this cannot be managed with ligamentous reconstruction.[21,22] Other SMO contraindications include neurovascular compromise, inflammatory joint disease, Charcot neuroarthropathy, acute or chronic infection, advanced tibiotalar joint (TTJ) disease, and advanced age. Smoking predisposes patients to the development of a nonunion; cessation is recommended.[21,22]

PREOPERATIVE RADIOGRAPHIC ASSESSMENT AND DEFORMITY ANALYSIS

Reviewing quality radiographs is crucial before considering SMO. Weight-bearing radiographs of anteroposterior, lateral, and mortise views of the ankle, as well as full-length radiographs, should be obtained to identify coexisting lower extremity deformities (**Fig. 1**).[23] The mechanical axis of the lower limb is defined as a line from the center of the femoral head to the center of the TTJ, and the anatomic axis of a bone is its mid-diaphyseal line.[24] The tibia's mechanical and anatomic axes are the same line,

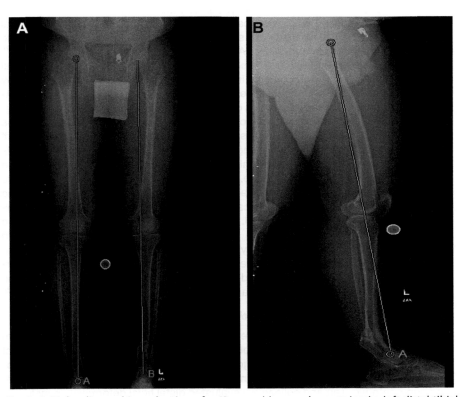

Fig. 1. Initial radiographic evaluation of a 42 year old man who sustained a left distal tibial fracture treated non-operatively. He presented to our clinic with ankle pain. (*A*) Full length standing anteroposterior view of bilateral views with normal mechanical axis deviation but with 2 cm of limb length discrepancy/shortening of the left side compared with the right lower extremity. There is also mild medial translation of the ankle joint. (*B*) Long leg lateral of the left lower extremity demonstrate 38° of recurvatum of the distal tibia without proximal deformity. There is a slight knee flexion contracture present. There is anterior ankle displacement with post-traumatic arthritis of the joint.

making it useful for preoperative planning. An ankle is in a neutral position with the tibial anatomic axis passing slightly lateral to the midsagittal plane of the ankle.[25]

Frontal plane deformities are characterized by varus or valgus malalignment of the distal tibia or ankle.[15] Measure this radiographically by examining the relationship between the calcaneus and the mid-diaphyseal line of the tibia. Typically, SMOs are performed when the apex of the deformity is at the ankle joint, yet the osteotomy is placed more proximally to correct it.[22] This will cause an angulation and translation effect of the osteotomy because it is proximal to the center of rotation of angulation (CORA).[22]

Valgus and Varus Ankles

In a valgus ankle, the reactive ground forces are laterally placed, making an increased load on the lateral aspect of the ankle joint.[11,15] This shifts the talus laterally into the fibula, causing syndesmosis distraction, sclerosis of the tibial plafond, distraction and stress of the distal tibiofibular joint, and articular destruction.[11,15,26] As the arthritic changes progress, the talus will continue to tilt in valgus, further causing incompetent medial soft tissue structures such as the deltoid ligament and the posterior tibial tendon.[26] Valgus ankle arthritis tends to progress much quicker than varus.[26,27] The lateral distal tibial angle (LDTA) will measure less than 86° in a valgus ankle; normal range is 86° to 92°.[15] The tibial articular surface (TAS) angle is defined by the anatomic tibial axis and the tibial plafond. If the TAS is greater than 90°, the ankle is in valgus.[28]

In a varus ankle, ground reactive forces are medially oriented. The broader medial malleolus articular surface offloads the increase in pressure, sparing the ankle initially from articular destruction.[15] Varus ankle deformity will develop from medial compartment overload that increases the stress on the underlying bone surface and with long-standing ankle varus, articular destruction will occur. In early stages of ankle varus, the TTJ is relatively neutral or in slight varus; however, in time, the talus will eventually tilt into varus, causing degenerative changes to the medial compartment.[27,29–35] This increased pressure will cause the medial talar shoulder to change into a more rounded shape with increased medial joint space. As the articular destruction progresses, there will also be increased stress on the medial soft tissues (ie, deltoid ligament and the posterior tibial tendon), subsequently causing contracture.[29] The lateral ligamentous structures become incompetent as well. Owing to lateral ligament failure and adaptive changes to the peroneal tendons, the talus will develop an anterolateral extrusion further defining severe varus deformity.[32,33] The varus ankle is more symptomatic due to an inability of the STJ to compensate as well in eversion as it does in inversion.[15] Therefore it is relevant to consider degenerative joint disease in the STJ. The LDTA measures greater than 92° in a varus ankle, and the TAS is lesser than 90°.[15,28]

Procurvatum and Recurvatum Deformities

Lateral ankle radiographs are imperative for determining the presence of procurvatum or recurvatum deformity in the sagittal plane.[4] The lateral talar process is a good point of reference for the center of ankle joint motion and should fall along the mid-diaphyseal line of the tibia. If there is anterior or posterior displacement, it is considered non-anatomic. Tarr and colleagues evaluated distal tibial deformities, concluding that sagittal plane deformities have the greatest increase in ankle joint contact pressures.[36] With 15° of anterior or posterior bowing, there is an increase of approximately 40% in uneven contact surface across the ankle joint.[31] The anatomic anterior distal tibial angle (ADTA) helps distinguish these deformities in the sagittal plane (normal range, 78°–82°).[15]

In procurvatum deformity, the ADTA will be greater than 82° and the radiographs will demonstrate a level of impingement of the TTJ anteriorly.[15] Distal tibial sagittal plane deformity is compensated by ankle dorsiflexion or plantarflexion. There is normally 50° of ankle plantarflexion and 20° of ankle dorsiflexion; owing to greater plantarflexion available, the foot will compensate for recurvatum much better than procurvatum. Typically, procurvatum deformity is more painful with limited compensation.[15] Despite more pain, the articular surface of the ankle joint is covered by the mortise.

In recurvatum deformity, the ADTA is lesser than 78° and the radiographs will demonstrate shearing forces because the tibia is oriented more posteriorly along the TTJ. Distal tibial recurvatum can be compensated by ankle plantarflexion as well as the triceps surae. In this deformity, the distal tibia CORA is displaced anteriorly which increases the anterior lever arm. Thus, a recurvatum deformity correction requires anterior translation.[15]

Plain radiography provides objective data for limb alignment and deformity. However, recent developments in three-dimensional (3D) models with weight-bearing computed tomography (WBCT) demonstrate high reliability for ankle OA and progressive pes plano valgus deformity.[37] Burssens and colleagues evaluated the effect of SMOs on ankle varus deformity and overall hindfoot alignment utilizing 3D measurements from WBCT. Their study found the SMO altered alignment by an average 2° to 3° compared with plain radiographs, concluding the benefit of WBCT in preoperative planning as well as postoperative evaluation.[37]

Combined single proton computed tomography and conventional computed tomography (SPECT/CT) provides a combination of metabolic and structural information of anatomy that recently expanded into preoperative planning for SMOs. Gross and colleagues investigated 85 preoperative SMOs with the SPECT/CT, concluding those with medial gutter activation had significantly worse preoperative American Orthopaedic Foot and Ankle Society (AOFAS) alignment scores, those with ankle valgus had worse AOFAS pain scores, and those with cystic lesions had worse Foot and Ankle Outcome Scores preoperatively. The study concluded that SPECT/CT was an effective prognostic indicator.[38]

SURGICAL TECHNIQUES

Patient positioning should allow for adequate exposure and access to the specific anatomy for the elected surgical approach. Approach should be based on osteotomy type with respect to local neurovascular, ligamentous, and tendinous structures.[15] When correcting in the frontal or sagittal plane, the surgeon should consider soft tissue releases for adequate deformity correction.[15] Patients are typically supine for an anterior incision, in a lateral decubitus or supine position with a bump under the ipsilateral hip for lateral approach, or supine with their knee bent and a bump under the ipsilateral calf for medial approach.[15]

The SMO is commonly performed in the metaphyseal zone to promote excellent healing in the distal tibia, whereas osteotomies made in the diaphysis may cause delayed healing.[15] Cutting bone with lower energy such as an osteotome can lead to faster healing compared with high-energy power tools that can cause thermal necrosis. If there are degenerative joint cases of the STJ, an STJ fusion may be indicated before the corrective osteotomy.

Valgus and Varus Ankles

For lateral soft tissue structures, testing the integrity of the anterior talofibular ligament and calcaneofibular ligament can aid in surgical repair or supplementation as well as any peroneal tendon debridement with tabularization, augmentation, or tenodesis.[27,32] For valgus ankle arthritis correction, a medial closing wedge SMO is utilized.

Under fluoroscopic guidance, K-wires are placed at the desired height with their intersection at the lateral cortex for the intended closing wedge. An anatomic T-plate is typically used with locking screws to the distal tibia, followed by osteotomy closure with compression. The plate is then fixed proximally, and final confirmation of correction is performed. A fibular osteotomy is also indicated—to prevent synostosis, this should be made either distal or proximal to the tibial osteotomy. The fibula is exposed through a longitudinal incision laterally. An oblique osteotomy is then made, and the fibula is gradually lengthened with a distractor. Once the desired length is achieved, the fibula is then fixated with a plate and screw construct.

Owing to contracture of the medial soft tissue structures with varus ankle, medial soft tissue release and prophylactic tarsal tunnel release are recommended.[39] For osseous correction of severe varus deformity of ankle arthritis, one may consider performing the SMO with either a medial opening wedge osteotomy or lateral closing wedge osteotomy.[7,27,34,35]

The medial open wedge osteotomy is performed commonly due to easy access to the distal medial aspect of the tibia. A medial longitudinal incision is made over the medial malleolus extending 10 to 12 cm proximally. The saphenous vein and nerve are carefully retracted with the skin flaps. The posterior tibial tendon is also carefully retracted posteriorly. The distal tibia is then exposed without excessive periosteal stripping. An oscillating saw is then used to make an oblique cut while preserving the lateral cortex to aid in stability of the wedge osteotomy. Next, a lamina spreader is used to pry open the wedge gently until the desired correction is obtained and confirmed under fluoroscopy. An appropriate-sized allograft is then placed, and a low-profile locking plate is placed medially to secure the correction. A fibular osteotomy is also performed at the same level as the opening medial wedge.[27,34,35]

The lateral closing wedge osteotomy is utilized in patients with compromised medial soft tissue. A 10 cm longitudinal incision is made just distal and anterior to the lateral malleolus. The distal tibia and fibula are exposed without excessive periosteal stripping. Once the distal syndesmosis is exposed, the proximal border will be utilized as a landmark for the fibular osteotomy height.[27,34,35] The wedge is created and the amount of shortening can be performed with either a simple bone block removal, Z-shaped osteotomy, or oblique wedge osteotomy. This is performed utilizing an oscillating saw with K-wires intersecting at the medial cortex to keep the medial hinge intact. Locking plate fixation is also placed laterally to secure the corrective osteotomy along with plate and screw fixation for the fibular osteotomy.[27,34,35]

Procurvatum and Recurvatum Deformities

An anterior approach is used for surgical correction of procurvatum. If length is needed, an acute opening wedge should be performed in conjunction with internal or external fixation with gradual opening wedge osteotomy and the apex of the wedge oriented posteriorly. If length is not indicated, an acute closing wedge osteotomy is performed.[15]

Regarding recurvatum, surgical correction may occur with an opening wedge, closing wedge, or focal dome osteotomy. Posterior osteotomies are difficult to perform technically due to soft tissue constraints; the anterior approach is recommended. If the osteotomy is away from the CORA, this will require secondary translation to allow for mechanical axis realignment.[15] If an opening wedge osteotomy is performed, the defect is filled with bone graft and secured with plates and screws. A closing wedge osteotomy typically will be fixated with plates, screws, or staples.

Focal dome osteotomies are utilized when the CORA is above the level of the ankle joint and can be performed either through an open or percutaneous approach.[15]

A percutaneous 3 cm stab incision can be performed either through an anterior or medial approach (**Figs. 2** and **3**). For the open approach, there should be adequate exposure of the tibia, with all neurovascular structures safely retracted out of the surgical field. Through the percutaneous approach, a single Schanz pin is placed central and parallel with the ankle joint both in the frontal and sagittal planes, and a series of drill holes are performed through the medial and lateral cortices with an osteotomy guide or a Rancho Cube (Smith and Nephew, Watford, UK). The osteotomy is then completed with a through-and-through osteotomy under fluoroscopic guidance. A fibular osteotomy is also performed either at the same level or distal to the tibial osteotomy through a small incision with multiple drill holes and a 1.8 mm Ilizarov wire. Next, a small Hoke osteotome is used to finalize the through-and-through osteotomy. The deformity is then reduced and fixated with fluoroscopy to confirm neutral anatomic alignment and correction along the mechanical axis.[15]

STAGING CORRECTIVE OSTEOTOMIES

TAA and ankle arthrodesis are surgical management options for end-stage ankle arthritis. Successful realignment of the ankle joint, particularly as it pertains to joint replacement, is critically important to ensure the longevity of the prosthesis.[40–43] Malalignment of the ankle joint with TAA increases edge forces, subsequently increasing risk of revisional surgery.[40–43] Coetzee reported 50% failure of total ankle replacements in patients with varus deformity greater than 20°.[17] It is vital to identify whether the deformity is intra-articular or extra-articular as a TAA alone may not be sufficient to correct the deformity. The importance of deformity correction before TAA has been discussed in the literature, noting that implant survivorship decreases with greater than 10° of coronal plane deformity.[18,44] It is preferable to perform coronal realignment simultaneously with TAA; however, complex deformity with adjunctive procedures will require a staged approach.[18,44]

In a study published by Knupp and colleagues, 16 patients with asymmetric end-stage ankle arthritis underwent simultaneous TAA and SMO. The authors reported improved outcomes and pain score reports, although 25% of patients required

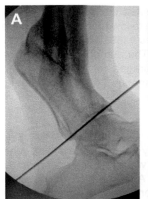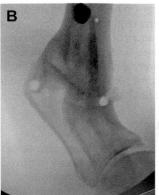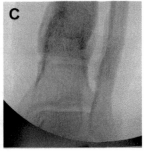

Fig. 2. Demonstrate intra-operative fluoroscopy with supramalleolar osteotomy of the tibia and fibula. (*A*) We identified and marked the ankle joint line intra-operatively along with the knee joint and mid-diaphyseal line of the tibia. (*B*) Multiple drill hole focal dome SMO was performed with a rancho cube approximately 3 cm from the ankle joint. (*C*) Intra-operative image depicting completion of focal dome osteotomy of the distal tibia.

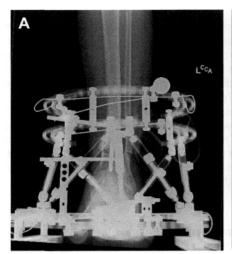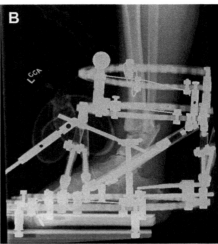

Fig. 3. (*A*) Antero-posterior (AP) weight-bearing radiograph status post distal tibial and fibular supramalleolar focal dome osteotomy through a minimally invasive technique with application of multiplanar external fixator. The senior author also performed a minimally invasive prophylactic tarsal tunnel release and posterior capulotomy with flexor tendon lengthening. (*B*) Lateral weight-bearing radiograph status post distal tibial and fibular supramalleolar osteotomy with application of multiplanar external fixator.

revisional surgery at short-term follow-up.[19] Deformities such as genu varum or valgum or limb length discrepancies due to growth arrest or trauma along the tibia may not be beneficial for simultaneous procedure; a staged approach may be better suited for these cases before TAA.[19]

Successful TAA with deformity should result in obtaining neutral ankle alignment for the implant, as well as a plantigrade and stable foot. To accomplish this before the TAA, the surgeon should achieve optimal alignment, ligamentous balancing, muscle–tendon balancing, and osseous realignment with a corrective SMO. A retrospective study performed by Day and colleagues evaluated and treated 8 patients with end-stage ankle OA with staged deformity correction followed by TAA.[41] Their results demonstrated improved patient-reported outcomes with successful deformity correction and minimal postoperative complications.[41] The authors concluded that with a staged approach, early weight-bearing is encouraged for bone healing for extra-articular osteotomy correction—whereas if simultaneous TAA was performed, early weight-bearing would not be possible.[41]

POSTOPERATIVE CONSIDERATIONS

Patients are non-weight-bearing immediately after surgery and placed in a thick Jones compression dressing. A drain is used, typically removed within the first postoperative day. Suture removal occurs between 2 and 3 weeks.[45] After the first postoperative visit, patients are placed in a non-weight-bearing cast for 6 to 8 weeks until there is evidence of radiographic osseous union on radiographs. Patients are gradually transitioned to weight-bearing in a walking boot and a rehabilitation program. Functional rehabilitation includes patient gait, progressive strengthening, proprioception, and range of motion. Full osseous union typically is achieved between 3 and 6 months, with full return to activity within 6 to 12 months (**Figs. 4** and **5**).[45]

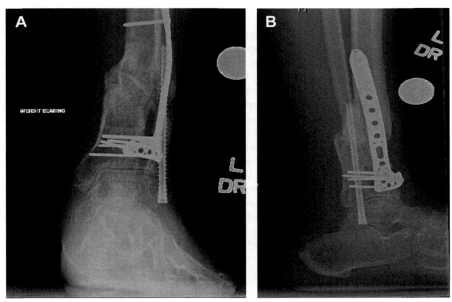

Fig. 4. (*A*) AP weight-bearing radiograph 6 months status post from initial surgery. Patient returned to the operating room April 2022 for external fixator removal with ORIF of distal SMO. Patient achieve full osseous consolidation osteotomy site 3 months post-op. (*B*) Lateral weight-bearing radiograph demonstrating significant improvement of distal tibial recurvatum with osseous consolidation of the osteotomy site.

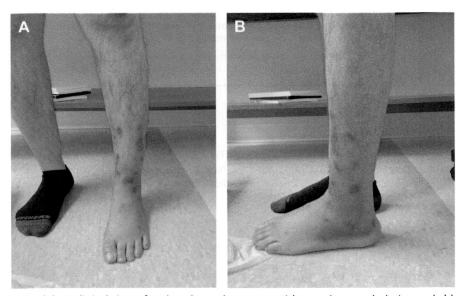

Fig. 5. (*A*) AP clinical view of patient 6 months post-op with no pain on ambulation and able to walk without assistive devices. Foot and leg are rectus. (*B*) Lateral view of the left lower extremity with rectus alignment of the foot and leg.

SUMMARY

Ankle OA can lead to wear of the articular surface of the joint and progressive degenerative changes.[45,46] Joint-preserving techniques such as the SMO can address deformities of the distal tibia and ankle joint to restore normal mechanics to the foot and ankle. This is achieved by shifting the center of force and reducing peak pressures within the ankle joint.[46,47] Realignment of the ankle joint may prevent or slow the progression of end-stage ankle arthritis and improve overall patient function. Different approaches and techniques are utilized to correct varus, valgus, procurvatum, and recurvatum deformities of the distal tibia. Fixation methods vary, including gradual or acute correction and internal or external fixation. The SMO can also be used in a staged approach in preparation for a TAA to optimize the implant's longevity and improve overall functional outcomes. When paired with a comprehensive understanding of deformity correction and a complete clinical and radiographic assessment, the SMO becomes a diverse and effective solution for joint preservation in the armamentarium of the orthopedic surgeon. Meticulous preoperative planning and precise surgical execution are necessary for the optimal patient outcome. The use of advanced technology such as WBCT and SPECT/CT can provide additional information for further preoperative planning.

CLINICS CARE POINTS

- Combined SPECT/CT and WBCT adds benefit with preoperative planning as well as postoperative evaluation for SMOs.
- Patient positioning should allow for adequate exposure and access to the specific anatomy for the elected surgical approach.
- The SMO is commonly performed in the metaphyseal zone to promote excellent healing in the distal tibia, whereas osteotomies made in the diaphysis may cause delayed healing.
- Corrective SMO prior to a TAA can achieve optimal osseous alignment of the ankle joint to prevent increases edge forces, subsequently increasing risk of revisional surgery.
- Staging TAA with SMOs may allow for early weight-bearing encourage bone healing, whereas if simultaneous TAA was performed, early weight-bearing would not be possible.

DISCLOSURES

N.A. Siddiqui is a consultant for Arthrex. The following organizations supported the institution of SM and NAS: DePuy Synthes, NuVasive Specialized Orthopedics, Orthofix, OrthoPediatrics, Paragon 28, Pega Medical, Smith & Nephew, Stryker, Turner Imaging Systems, and WishBone Medical.

ACKNOWLEDGMENTS

The authors thank Robert P. Farley, BS, for his assistance with this article.

REFERENCES

1. Delco ML, Kennedy JG, Bonassar LJ, et al. Post-traumatic osteoarthritis of the ankle: a distinct clinical entity requiring new research approaches. J Orthop Res 2017;35(3):440–53.

2. Anderson MR, Houck JR, Saltzman CL, et al. Validation and generalizability of preoperative PROMIS scores to predict postoperative success in foot and ankle patients. Foot Ankle Int 2018;39(7):763–70.
3. Peyron JG. The epidemiology of osteoarthritis. In: Moskowitz RW, Howell DS, Goldberg VM, et al, editors. Osteoarthritis: diagnosis and treatment. Philadelphia, PA: WB Saunders; 1984. p. 9–27.
4. Ankle and foot considerations. In: Paley D, Herzenberg JE, editors. Principles of deformity correction. Berlin, Germany: Springer-Verlag; 2002. p. 571–645.
5. Horisberger M, Valderrabano V, Hintermann B. Posttraumatic ankle osteoarthritis after ankle-related fractures. J Orthop Trauma 2009;23(1):60–7.
6. Nuesch C, Huber C, Paul J, et al. Mid- to long-term clinical outcome and gait biomechanics after realignment surgery in asymmetric ankle osteoarthritis. Foot Ankle Int 2015;36(8):908–18.
7. Siddiqui NA, Millonig KJ. Foot and ankle deformity analysis and surgical planning. In: Standard SC, Herzenberg JE, editors. The art of limb alignment. 11th edition. Baltimore, MD: Rubin Institute of Advanced Orthopedics, Sinai Hospital of Baltimore; 2022. p. 283–305.
8. Lloyd J, Elsayed S, Hariharan K, et al. Revisiting the concept of talar shift in ankle fractures. Foot Ankle Int 2006;27(10):793–6.
9. Kimizuka M, Kurosawa H, Fukubayashi T. Load-bearing pattern of the ankle joint: contact area and pressure distribution. Arch Orthop Trauma Surg 1980;96(1):45–9.
10. Thomas RH, Daniels TR. Ankle arthritis. J Bone Joint Surg Am 2003;85(5):923–36.
11. Ramsey PL, Hamilton W. Changes in tibiotalar area of contact caused by lateral talar shift. J Bone Joint Surg Am 1976;58(3):356–7.
12. Stamatis ED, Cooper PS, Myerson MS. Supramalleolar osteotomy for the treatment of distal tibial angular deformities and arthritis of the ankle joint. Foot Ankle Int 2003;24(10):754–64.
13. Barg A, Pagenstert GI, Horisberger M, et al. Supramalleolar osteotomies for degenerative joint disease of the ankle joint: indication, technique and results. Int Orthop 2013;37(9):1683–95.
14. Barg A, Saltzman CL. Single-stage supramalleolar osteotomy for coronal plane deformity. Curr Rev Musculoskelet Med 2014;7(4):277–91.
15. Siddiqui NA, Herzenberg JE, Lamm BM. Supramalleolar osteotomy for realignment of the ankle joint. Clin Podiatr Med Surg 2012;29(4):465–82.
16. Pagenstert GI, Hintermann B, Barg A, et al. Realignment surgery as alternative treatment of varus and valgus ankle osteoarthritis. Clin Orthop Relat Res 2007;462:156–68.
17. Coetzee JC. Management of varus or valgus ankle deformity with ankle replacement. Foot Ankle Clin 2008;13(3):509–20.
18. Gauvain TT, Hames MA, McGarvey WC. Malalignment correction of the lower limb before, during, and after total ankle arthroplasty. Foot Ankle Clin 2017;22(2):311–39.
19. Knupp M, Stufkens SA, Bolliger L, et al. Total ankle replacement and supramalleolar steotomies for malaligned osteoarthritic ankles. Tech Foot Ankle Surg 2010;9(4):175–81.
20. Knupp M, Pagenstert G, Valderrabano V, et al. Osteotomies in varus malalignment of the ankle. Operat Orthop Traumatol 2008;20(3):262–73.
21. Pagenstert G, Knupp M, Valderrabano V, et al. Realignment surgery for valgus ankle osteoarthritis. Operat Orthop Traumatol 2009;21(1):77–87.

22. Colin F, Gaudot F, Odri G, et al. Supramalleolar osteotomy: techniques, indications and outcomes in a series of 83 cases. Orthop Traumatol Surg Res 2014; 100(4):413–8.
23. Lamm BM, Siddiqui NA. Obtaining x-rays of the ankle and foot for deformity analysis. In: Standard SC, Herzenberg JE, editors. The art of limb alignment. 11th ed. Baltimore, MD: Rubin Institute of Advanced Orthopedics, Sinai Hospital of Baltimore; 2022. p. 59–72.
24. Standard SC. Normal limb alignment. In: Standard SC, Herzenberg JE, editors. The art of limb alignment. 11th ed. Baltimore, MD: Rubin Institute of Advanced Orthopedics, Sinai Hospital of Baltimore; 2022. p. 1–2.
25. Lamm BM, Siddiqui NA. Foot and ankle: normal alignment. In: Standard SC, Herzenberg JE, editors. The art of limb alignment. 11th ed. Baltimore, MD: Rubin Institute of Advanced Orthopedics, Sinai Hospital of Baltimore; 2022. p. 261–8.
26. Krähenbühl N, Susdorf R, Barg A, et al. Supramalleolar osteotomy in post-traumatic valgus ankle osteoarthritis. Int Orthop 2020;44(3):535–43.
27. Zhao HM, Wen XD, Zhang Y, et al. Supramalleolar osteotomy with medial distraction arthroplasty for ankle osteoarthritis with talar tilt. J Orthop Surg Res 2019; 14(1):120.
28. Hintermann B, Knupp M, Barg A. Supramalleolar osteotomies for the treatment of ankle arthritis. J Am Acad Orthop Surg 2016;24(7):424–32.
29. Harstall R, Lehmann O, Krause F, et al. Supramalleolar lateral closing wedge osteotomy for the treatment of varus ankle arthrosis. Foot Ankle Int 2007;28(5): 542–8.
30. Lee WC, Moon JS, Lee K, et al. Indications for supramalleolar osteotomy in patients with ankle osteoarthritis and varus deformity. J Bone Joint Surg Am 2011; 93(13):1243–8.
31. Takakura Y, Takaoka T, Tanaka Y, et al. Results of opening-wedge osteotomy for the treatment of a post-traumatic varus deformity of the ankle. J Bone Joint Surg Am 1998;80(2):213–8.
32. Lacorda JB, Jung HG, Im JM. Supramalleolar distal tibiofibular osteotomy for medial ankle osteoarthritis: current concepts. Clin Orthop Surg 2020;12(3):271–8.
33. Rush SM. Supramalleolar osteotomy. Clin Podiatr Med Surg 2009;26(2):245–57.
34. Krähenbühl N, Akkaya M, Deforth M, et al. Extraarticular supramalleolar osteotomy in asymmetric varus ankle osteoarthritis. Foot Ankle Int 2019;40(8):936–47.
35. Lee WC. Extraarticular supramalleolar osteotomy for managing varus ankle osteoarthritis, alternatives for osteotomy: How and why? Foot Ankle Clin 2016;21(1): 27–35.
36. Tarr RR, Resnick CT, Wagner KS, et al. Changes in tibiotalar joint contact areas following experimentally induced tibial angular deformities. Clin Orthop Relat Res 1985;199:72–80.
37. Burssens A, Susdorf R, Krähenbühl N, et al. Supramalleolar osteotomy for ankle varus deformity alters subtalar joint alignment. Foot Ankle Int 2022. https://doi.org/10.1177/10711007221108097.
38. Gross CE, Barfield W, Schqeizer C, et al. The utility of the ankle SPECT/CT scan to predict functional and clinical outcomes in supramalleolar osteotomy patients. J Orthop Res 2018;36:2015–21.
39. Lamm BM, Paley D, Testani M, et al. Tarsal tunnel decompression in leg lengthening and deformity correction of the foot and ankle. J Foot Ankle Surg 2007; 46(3):201–6.

40. Deforth M, Krähenbühl N, Zwicky L, et al. Supramalleolar osteotomy for tibial component malposition in total ankle replacement. Foot Ankle Int 2017;38(9): 952–6.
41. Day J, Principe PS, Caolo KC, et al. A staged approach to combined extra-articular limb deformity correction and total ankle arthroplasty for end-stage ankle arthritis. Foot Ankle Int 2021;42(3):257–67.
42. Doets HC, Brand R, Nelissen RG. Total ankle arthroplasty in inflammatory joint disease with use of two mobile-bearing designs. J Bone Joint Surg Am 2006; 88(6):1272–84.
43. Escudero MI, Le V, Barahona M, et al. Total ankle arthroplasty survival and risk factors for failure. Foot Ankle Int 2019;40(9):997–1006.
44. Kim BS, Choi WJ, Kim YS, et al. Total ankle replacement in moderate to severe varus deformity of the ankle. J Bone Joint Surg Br 2009;91(9):1183–90.
45. Mulhern JL, Protzman NM, Brigido SA, et al. Supramalleolar osteotomy: indications and surgical techniques. Clin Podiatr Med Surg 2015;32(3):445–61.
46. Koo JW, Park SH, Kim KC, et al. The preliminary report about the modified supramalleolar tibial osteotomy for asymmetric ankle osteoarthritis. J Orthop Surg 2019;27(1). 2309499019829204.
47. Kim J, Henry JK, Kim JB, et al. Dome supramalleolar osteotomies for the treatment of ankle pain with opposing coronal plane deformities between ankle and the lower limb. Foot Ankle Int 2022;43(4):474–85.

UNITED STATES POSTAL SERVICE® Statement of Ownership, Management, and Circulation (All Periodicals Publications Except Requester Publications)

1. Publication Title	2. Publication Number	3. Filing Date
CLINICS IN PODIATRIC MEDICINE & SURGERY	000 – 707	9/18/2023

4. Issue Frequency	5. Number of Issues Published Annually	6. Annual Subscription Price
JAN, APR, JUL, OCT	4	$329

7. Complete Mailing Address of Known Office of Publication (Not printer) (Street, city, county, state, and ZIP+4®)

ELSEVIER INC.
230 Park Avenue, Suite 800
New York, NY 10169

Contact Person: Malathi Samayan
Telephone (Include area code): 91-44-4299-4507

8. Complete Mailing Address of Headquarters or General Business Office of Publisher (Not printer)

ELSEVIER INC.
230 Park Avenue, Suite 800
New York, NY 10169

9. Full Names and Complete Mailing Addresses of Publisher, Editor, and Managing Editor (Do not leave blank)

Publisher (Name and complete mailing address)

Dolores Meloni, ELSEVIER INC.
1600 JOHN F KENNEDY BLVD. SUITE 1600
PHILADELPHIA, PA 19103-2899

Editor (Name and complete mailing address)

Megan Ashdown, ELSEVIER INC.
1600 JOHN F KENNEDY BLVD. SUITE 1600
PHILADELPHIA, PA 19103-2899

Managing Editor (Name and complete mailing address)

PATRICK MANLEY, ELSEVIER INC.
1600 JOHN F KENNEDY BLVD. SUITE 1600
PHILADELPHIA, PA 19103-2899

10. Owner (Do not leave blank. If the publication is owned by a corporation, give the name and address of the corporation immediately followed by the names and addresses of all stockholders owning or holding 1 percent or more of the total amount of stock. If not owned by a corporation, give the names and addresses of the individual owners. If owned by a partnership or other unincorporated firm, give its name and address as well as those of each individual owner. If the publication is published by a nonprofit organization, give its name and address.)

Full Name	Complete Mailing Address
WHOLLY OWNED SUBSIDIARY OF REED/ELSEVIER, US HOLDINGS	1600 JOHN F KENNEDY BLVD. SUITE 1600 PHILADELPHIA, PA 19103-2899

11. Known Bondholders, Mortgagees, and Other Security Holders Owning or Holding 1 Percent or More of Total Amount of Bonds, Mortgages, or Other Securities. If none, check box ▶ ☐ None

Full Name	Complete Mailing Address
N/A	

12. Tax Status (For completion by nonprofit organizations authorized to mail at nonprofit rates) (Check one)
The purpose, function, and nonprofit status of this organization and the exempt status for federal income tax purposes:
☒ Has Not Changed During Preceding 12 Months
☐ Has Changed During Preceding 12 Months (Publisher must submit explanation of change with this statement)

PS Form 3526, July 2014 [Page 1 of 4 (see instructions page 4)] PSN: 7530-01-000-9931 PRIVACY NOTICE: See our privacy policy on www.usps.com

---

13. Publication Title	14. Issue Date for Circulation Data Below
CLINICS IN PODIATRIC MEDICINE & SURGERY	JULY 2023

15. Extent and Nature of Circulation

		Average No. Copies Each Issue During Preceding 12 Months	No. Copies of Single Issue Published Nearest to Filing Date
a. Total Number of Copies (Net press run)		132	133
b. Paid Circulation (By Mail and Outside the Mail)	(1) Mailed Outside-County Paid Subscriptions Stated on PS Form 3541 (Include paid distribution above nominal rate, advertiser's proof copies, and exchange copies)	91	93
	(2) Mailed In-County Paid Subscriptions Stated on PS Form 3541 (Include paid distribution above nominal rate, advertiser's proof copies, and exchange copies)	0	0
	(3) Paid Distribution Outside the Mails Including Sales Through Dealers and Carriers, Street Vendors, Counter Sales, and Other Paid Distribution Outside USPS®	11	10
	(4) Paid Distribution by Other Classes of Mail Through the USPS (e.g., First-Class Mail®)	6	6
c. Total Paid Distribution (Sum of 15b (1), (2), (3), and (4))		108	109
d. Free or Nominal Rate Distribution (By Mail and Outside the Mail)	(1) Free or Nominal Rate Outside-County Copies included on PS Form 3541	23	23
	(2) Free or Nominal Rate In-County Copies Included on PS Form 3541	0	0
	(3) Free or Nominal Rate Copies Mailed at Other Classes Through the USPS (e.g., First-Class Mail)	0	0
	(4) Free or Nominal Rate Distribution Outside the Mail (Carriers or other means)	1	1
e. Total Free or Nominal Rate Distribution (Sum of 15d (1), (2), (3) and (4))		24	24
f. Total Distribution (Sum of 15c and 15e)		132	133
g. Copies not Distributed (See Instructions to Publishers #4 (page 43))		0	0
h. Total (Sum of 15f and g)		132	133
i. Percent Paid (15c divided by 15f times 100)		81.47%	81.95%

* If you are claiming electronic copies, go to line 16 on page 3. If you are not claiming electronic copies, skip to line 17 on page 3.

PS Form 3526, July 2014 (Page 2 of 4)

16. Electronic Copy Circulation

	Average No. Copies Each Issue During Preceding 12 Months	No. Copies of Single Issue Published Nearest to Filing Date
a. Paid Electronic Copies	▶	
b. Total Paid Print Copies (Line 15c) + Paid Electronic Copies (Line 16a)	▶	
c. Total Print Distribution (Line 15f) + Paid Electronic Copies (Line 16a)	▶	
d. Percent Paid (Both Print & Electronic Copies) (16b divided by 16c × 100)	▶	

☒ I certify that 50% of all my distributed copies (electronic and print) are paid above a nominal price.

17. Publication of Statement of Ownership

☒ If the publication is a general publication, publication of this statement is required. Will be printed in the OCTOBER 2023 issue of this publication. ☐ Publication not required.

18. Signature and Title of Editor, Publisher, Business Manager, or Owner

Malathi Samayan

Malathi Samayan - Distribution Controller

Date 9/18/2023

I certify that all information furnished on this form is true and complete. I understand that anyone who furnishes false or misleading information on this form or who omits material or information requested on the form may be subject to criminal sanctions (including fines and imprisonment) and/or civil sanctions (including civil penalties).

PS Form 3526, July 2014 (Page 3 of 4) PRIVACY NOTICE: See our privacy policy on www.usps.com

9780443182341